Psychoanalytic Work with Children in Hospital

Psychoanalytic Work with Children in Hospital presents the experiences of a psychoanalyst working within a hospital paediatric department.

It explores the possibilities for applying psychoanalytic theory when working with children in hospital and how it can be extended to include parents, caregivers, health care staff and volunteers. Each chapter of the book addresses an issue or area of professional experience that presented Franco D'Alberton with clinical or technical questions, outlining the core concern and then exploring his attempt to provide answers to these questions. This volume presents many possible applications of psychoanalytic theory in a paediatric hospital, encompassing issues encountered by health care staff and volunteers as well as by parents and their hospitalized children, such as physical pain, meetings and information sharing and group settings. It also describes therapeutic interventions directed toward both children and parents.

This book will be key reading for child and adolescent psychoanalysts, psychotherapists, and clinical psychologists in practice and in training. It will also interest clinicians seeking to understand how psychoanalytic work can be applied in hospital and health care settings.

Franco D'Alberton is a child and adolescent psychoanalyst, and a member of the Italian Psychoanalytic Society and the International Psychoanalytic Association.

Psychoanalytic Work with Children in Hospital

Franco D'Alberton

Translated by Gina Atkinson

Routledge
Taylor & Francis Group

LONDON AND NEW YORK

Designed cover image: Malufatti, Souls, 2017

First published in English 2023
by Routledge
4 Park Square, Milton Park, Abingdon, Oxon OX14 4RN

and by Routledge
605 Third Avenue, New York, NY 10158

Routledge is an imprint of the Taylor & Francis Group, an informa business

© 2023 Franco D'Alberton
Translated by Gina Atkinson

Published in Italian by Milano: Franco Angeli Editore 2018

British Library Cataloguing-in-Publication Data
A catalogue record for this book is available from the British Library

ISBN: 978-1-032-17201-9 (hbk)
ISBN: 978-1-032-17202-6 (pbk)
ISBN: 978-1-003-25223-8 (ebk)

DOI: 10.4324/9781003252238

Typeset in Times New Roman
by Apex CoVantage, LLC

Contents

13 Group Sessions with Volunteers: On Books and Reading
    in the Hospital   204

    Concluding Reflections   215

    Index   217

Preface – By Stefano Bolognini[1]

It is a particular pleasure for me to present this book and to bring the reader into contact with its author, his narrations, his reflections, his competence, and with the many things that – from an expert psychoanalyst, committed to paediatrics for many years – he has known live, studied seriously, and co-participated in with passion, sharing his expertise with teachers, colleagues, and students in the broader environment of hospital institutions.

I have known Franco D'Alberton for a long time and I have had occasion to appreciate his humane generosity, his lively scientific curiosity, his acute mode of clinical observation, and his particular disposition (which not everyone has) toward valuing professional investment in the social – not in a generically political sense, that is – but in actuality, on the level of daily communal responsibility.

This book, which provides an important scientific contribution to a very thorough understanding of children's psychic reality, of their families and caregivers, when all these subjectivities (often partially and painfully outside awareness) are encountered in the hospital setting, is also the author's act of sensitive yet authoritative testimony around what is still to be understood and to be transformed within that providential, ultra-necessary institution – in that place where everything seems to be "logical" enough, in a complex way and from a functional point of view but is still not very "psychological" with respect to the extremely important perception of individuals' experiences and of the complexity of their internal lives and relationships – both those of patients and their families and of professional groups who interact with them, beginning with the first request for help and on through diagnosis, outpatient assistance, and eventual hospitalization, for the most diverse pathologies.

The first thing to be clarified in order to dispel possible misunderstandings is that this text does not contain generically supportive suggestions along the lines of "be kind, welcoming, and benevolent."

D'Alberton's well-documented and in-depth research and reflections in the book's clinical sections are supported by a refined, up-to-date, theoretical-technical competence, the product not only of his specialized reading and undoubtedly mature professional experience directly in the field but also and especially of his consistent following of organized national and international scientific activities in the psychoanalytic community, in which he has for years played an active role with his papers, discussions with colleagues and interactive exchanges at various levels.

Having had occasion to systematically attend, for professional reasons, nearly all the major international psychoanalytic conferences of the past twenty years, I can bear witness to the fact that almost always I had the pleasure not only of meeting up with Franco but also of seeing him committed and involved in a truly passionate way in working groups and in theoretical-clinical debates, knowing that he was dedicated to importing into the work environment (either the hospital or the analytic office) what he had learned or simply what had absorbed him in those enriching forums.

Franco defines himself, in an early chapter of the book, as "a psychoanalyst who played away from home" – referring to his hospital work carried out primarily in the mornings, at best putting together "two roles that I tried equally hard to keep together: a psychoanalyst's activity in my office and that of a psychologist in the hospital."

In my view, he has succeeded very well.

This has definitely been an integrative book, one of connections and of difficult and complex harmonization, certainly, as my colleagues well know (a minority today, among analysts; at one time it wasn't so) who inhabit two distinct professional arenas: the psychoanalytic one and the psychiatric or paediatric one or that of other medical branches in the hospital setting.

In Italy, we have had a long and prestigious tradition of psychoanalysts committed to psychiatry, in the child neuropsychiatric field and in social services assisting couples and families (primarily as consultants), and less so in the hospital paediatric environment, where the analyst's function-bridge – or at any rate, that of the analytically trained therapist – initially seems less clear or less obvious not only to users (to young patients and especially their families) but also to many doctors and to the hospital staff.

D'Alberton says:

> The medical culture and the psychoanalytic culture are both, in some ways, jealously possessive of their own scientific-cultural arenas and of their own interventional tools: they enjoy reciprocal respect as long as "each keeps to its own." But how does one distinguish the respective areas of intervention when faced with a newborn who has been in an incubator for a few days?
>
> [p. 5]

Things have gradually changed over the years, and that's due precisely to the work, the passion, and at times the true institutional resilience of therapists who have known how to advocate for – and then to protect – an integrative reading of the psychic dimension in settings where the psychic seems to be essentially denied, repressed, split, or at least ignored and eluded. Often, diffuse anxieties of illness and death are so strong as to make everyone, both caregivers and patients, hyperdefensive, armoured and anesthetized to the point of an erasure of subjectivity, in the name of a stringent objectivity that should be very effective and prevalent in order to justify every anti-psychic deviation in relationships with the patient and the family. In such settings, institutional resistances tend to cast the very presence of the psychic (and those who work with it) as a pathological anomaly in itself – a dysfunctional symptom, a "foreign body."

The attentive reader will find in this book the patient, perspicacious revelation – at times obvious but more often veiled – of deep and powerful trans-psychic structures that exist among young patients, parents, and caregivers: transferential reactivations of contents, of ghosts and of defences that circulate unrecognized even in intra-hospital contact.

On top of collective anxiety defences, one must also add – even though times have changed, fortunately, in relation to the past, at least somewhat – the persistence of a certain mentality in which "referring to the patient's individuality, investigating the world of his affects and connections, has become a sort of luxury" (p. 6–7), rather than as a difficult but potentially extremely valuable means of accessing internal factors that influence the subject's quality of life, his attitude regarding illness, his collaboration with caregivers, and at times even the clinical course of certain complex vicissitudes.

And if, from the medical side, the analyst is destined almost by fiat to encounter difficulties and resistances to his type of approach and investigation, on the other hand, on the psychoanalytic side, he will have to view the situation with residual scepticism that derives not only from the more traditional sectors of his armamentarium but also from his internal state, from the subtly tormenting, more purist-oriented and rigid "friendly fire" of his superego and ego ideal:

> When I began to work in the hospital, it seemed to me I was led back to golden analytic currency to be spent in clinical work – coins that I had put aside over long years of analysis and training, but that . . . didn't seem to be the currency in use in the "hospital" territory. Expecting that the conditions would be created in which this currency could be used, I went around with these coins in my pocket, exchanging one now and then for a coin that purists would define as the up-to-date, bronze currency.
>
> [p. 8]

I think that one could not describe any better than this the delicate and difficult work of mediation and connection between these different clinical-cultural worlds, in which "the analyst away from home" is put to the test from both sides and must have great trust in his own intelligence and sensitivity in order to utilize his competence and skills in a way that – to continue the metaphor – is effectively "spendable."

And besides, in that bronze currency, in that apparently humble capacity to communicate with patients and their families "in plain language" ("Doctor, say it to me in plain language" was a frequent request to Dr D'Alberton in conversations with persons to whom he had described their condition in exemplary but incomprehensible scientific terms), there can be a real treasure, if the analyst has the ability, willingness, and also the inclination to truly get in tune with the patient's experience.

I don't intend to take up too much space between the author's discussion and his readers.

If as a colleague, I can happily congratulate Franco D'Alberton for the scientifically rich, mature, and agreeable level of this book, then as an ordinary (but resonant) reader, I can announce in advance to other readers that in these pages they will find – alongside theoretical sections – many clinical stories that are extremely touching for their deep explorations and many very effective "cross-sections" of inner reflection, which reveal a psychoanalyst at work even "without the couch" – including many of his personal, intimate, and always relevant thoughts about an experiential field shared with patients, their families, and colleagues but undoubtedly drawn from the sincerest depths of the psychoanalyst as a human being.

Note

1   IPA (International Psychoanalytic Association) past President.

Acknowledgments

This book describes a journey of many years in a paediatric hospital setting, and it represents an attempt to respond to questions that clinical demands have triggered in fields in which not many well-established experiences are available.

These have been intense and stimulating years in which I have had contact with people of great human and professional depth and rigor, who gave me the opportunity to experiment in fields that I didn't know very well. From many of these people, I learned a great deal: from doctors, psychology colleagues, nurses, social workers and patients.

I'd like to especially thank Professor Cicognani, director of what was then called the Pediatric and Endocrinological Pediatric Ward of Sant'Orsola-Malpighi Bologna University Hospital. Professor Cicognani was the first to believe in the spirit that animated the experiences I will describe, whose operations were then followed by Professors Pirazzoli, Bernardi and Mazzanti. I have enormous gratitude to them for the realm of work that we carried out together, as well as to Professor Fernando Maria Picchio, Marco Bonvicini and Gaetano Gargiulo of the Cardiology and Cardiosurgical Unit and to Professor Cristina Meriggiola of the unit specializing in gynaecology and the physiopathology of human reproduction.

Professor Salardi, together with Alessandra Cassio, were equally involved and enthusiastically supportive of the various projects. Other competent and steadfast companions along this journey were Rosalba Bergamaschi, Davide Tassinari, Franco Zappulla, Stefano Zucchini, Andrea Pasini, Salvatore Cazzato, Federico Baronio, Ilaria Bettocchi, Milva Bal, Monia Gennari, Ilaria Corsini, Sara Forti, Manuela Scarano, Maria Perri, Giulio Maltoni, Rita Ortolano and Federica Tamburino.

With Antonio Balsamo, sharing the most careful and accurate work in the field of variations of sexual differentiation led to an especially productive collaboration and to joint participation in many experiences in this field, both nationally and internationally.

To Manuela Mancini, Virginia Lepore, Barbara Martelli and to all the nurses and social workers with whom I was in contact, I must express great appreciation for their professionalism and their invaluable work that goes on every day, silently and generously.

To the group of psychology colleagues with whom, over time, I shared the experiences that this book is about, I offer particular thanks for having allowed me to experience the beauty and pleasure of helping with the birth and formation of ideas within a group's thinking.

A heartfelt thank you, then, to Laura Nardi, Maura Foresti, Graziana D'Addabbo, Nicoletta Bisacchi, Daniela Gaddoni, Catia Giovannini, Federica Stortoni, Chiara Ferracuti, Sofia Vissani, Delia Conte, Daniele Bilacchi, Marta Vimborsati, Sofia Palmeira, Giulia Nardacchione, Martina Prandi, Elisa Serra, Elisa Degli Esposti, Filippo Gibiino, Giulia Smargiacchi, Martina Rinaldi, Micol Natali, Maria Celeste Di Febbo and all the others who shared these experiences over time.

This book would not have been possible without the contribution of the people whom I met in the course of my professional activity; to them I extend deep thanks for having consented to the publication of clinical material, though anonymized and unrecognizable, that pertains to parts of their lives.

Some of the clinical material was presented on various occasions at the Società Italiana di Psicoanalisi, at SEPEA (Société Européenne pour la Psychanalyse de l'Enfant et de l'Adolescent), to ASUPEA (Association Suisse pour la Psychanalyse de l'Enfant et de l'Adolescent) and at EPF (European Psychoanalytic Federation), in meetings having to do with psychosomatics, adolescence and child analysis.

The material on functional disturbances and bodily expression was published in the *Rivista di Psicoanalisi* and the *Italian Psychoanalytic Annual*, whose editors I thank for their consent to its publication here.

Valentina Misgur and Silvia Brizio have played an extremely valuable role in editing the book in Italian and Anna Maria Roda in supporting it.

And last but not least, coming to this English edition, a warm grateful thank you to Gina Atkinson for her patient and supportive work of translation and editing.

To those and to many others whom I can't cite, I extend my deep gratitude.

Introduction

> We must presume rather that the psychical trauma – or more precisely the memory of the trauma – acts like a foreign body.
>
> [Breuer and Freud 1893, p. 6]

The title of this book introduces the work of a psychoanalyst and his professional contacts with children, their parents, and health institutions – in particular, the hospital.

The metaphor of a foreign body cited in my epigraph, with its many possible meanings, seems to me a good starting point for this introduction. It appeared, almost on its own, in the course of a meeting with the parents of a ten-year-old girl, whom we will call Giulia, who suffered from a pronounced respiratory disturbance.

For two months, Giulia had had a persistent cough; every pharmacological treatment proved to be ineffective, and her paediatrician had advised hospitalization in order to check for the possible presence of a foreign body in the bronchial cavities.

Once she was on the ward, the pulmonologist, although observing an apparently organic symptomatology, had the feeling that something was missing from the picture and asked that I see the child to gather information about her emotional condition before an invasive examination took place to investigate the hypothesis of a foreign body.

From my first meeting with Giulia, it appeared with a certain clarity that the "foreign body" for this child was her own body, through which worries and fantasies about herself and her relationships with her parents found a means of expression. While she found herself at the dawning of the process of preadolescence, the relationship between her parents was on the edge of a breaking point. Giulia, who couldn't allow herself to represent to herself or to express her emotions in any other way, had unconsciously transformed those unthinkable feelings into a somatic symptom that impeded her respiratory processes. She tried to expel, to cough up a mental irritation – a blocked thought in relation to changes in her body and her mind pertaining to a possible separation of her parents. Her hospital

DOI: 10.4324/9781003252238-1

stay, on the other hand, slowed the disquieting tensions between autonomy and dependence, and her progress affected the decisions made by her parents, who, both seriously concerned about her condition, reached a new, temporary accord in staying close by in the hospital, day and night.

From the earliest history of psychoanalysis, the metaphor of a foreign body was used by Breuer and Freud (1893) to describe the action of trauma in the psychic apparatus and to make sense of defensive processes and symptomatic expressions that originated from it. A mental representation that was unacceptable to the subject resulted in the setting up of defensive mechanisms. At that time, it was thought that they consisted basically of repression, giving rise to the neurotic symptom as a compromise between instinctual desire and censorship, with the goal of keeping the traumatic memory out of consciousness.

There have been no great changes since then, when the body, which was recognized as a possible theatre of conflict between representations and internal frameworks, was seen to afford them a means of expression. Nonetheless, recent innovations in the neurosciences and in psychoanalysis have highlighted the influence of various early somatic and implicitly emotional experiences (Mancia 2004; Riolo 2009) that can determine deficits in symbolization and mental representation.

Psychoanalysis and the Hospital

In the multifaceted hospital culture, one sees an oscillation between an emphasis on the possible psychological influences in every somatic manifestation and the complementary devaluation that tends to take into account only "objective" criteria, expressed by the ever more refined medical techniques of exploitable investigation. It can happen that the body, probed in all its crevices and measured along every possible physiological variable, ends up being kept at a distance and considered foreign when it expresses signs rooted in a more intimate look at the meaning of the existential experience of each individual patient, "unfortunately" capable of slipping away from even the most refined technological instruments.

This book was born out of the experience of a psychoanalyst who played "away from home," "a psychoanalyst without a couch" (Racamier 1970), working as a psychologist in a university paediatric hospital, in the thousands of managerial and clinical activities that a structure of this type requires.

As is well known, psychoanalysis is the discipline that holds that an important part of people's psychic life unfolds beyond the conscious level and is located in an area that we are not aware of, one in which continuous movement occurs between somatic sensations, instinctual needs, fantasies, and desires. The development of a person through the point of expressing his own subjectivity depends on the cohesion of his ego and the balance that, in a given period of life, successfully arrives at the complex interrelationship among external reality, the needs of the drive, and the rules of the individual's own moral values, whether conscious or unconscious.

In the chapters that follow, we will see how, at times, emotional conflicts can seize the vehicle of the body and express themselves through somatic disturbances. Sometimes the presence of a physical malady can alter subtle emotional balances and determine the acceptance of treatment and the adaptation that the condition will ultimately permit.

The influence of the unconscious and of how little it can be grasped if one is focused only on the rationality and conscious thought of the people whom we meet can be appreciated by following the progress of a session with a 16-year-old girl. She was suffering from the onset of a pathology that required periodic check-ups and continual treatment in order to avoid relapses that occurred with a certain frequency. This girl was sent to see me because, in later adolescence, she had decided to resist the changes in her body, which she didn't like and which she attributed to a change in her treatment regimen. She had decided to stop eating, trying to reach an ideal weight that continually went down. Every argument by those who treated her ran up against an apparent rationality in her plan and intentions.

Naturally, she explained to me her opinion of how things were; her medical condition, worries about her health, and the unexpected exacerbations that had accompanied her since birth were irrelevant. It was her face that she didn't like – "swollen" by the medications she took, even though the dosages were lower now. Her adolescent body had become foreign, something to struggle against; she worried only about easily identifiable, superficial objectives, putting aside a deeper sense of foreignness that was too saturated with deep anxieties and feelings about death (Laufer 2005; Ruggiero 2016; Nicolò 2009; Goisis 2014).

She had a dream about being in Bologna, even though in the dream she was surrounded by buildings in a city near the one where she lived. She had to go eat at McDonalds with her father, crossing a bridge and passing by a monument where there was a famous person's tomb. Suddenly, she had the feeling of continuous falling, as though in a kind of videogame. The third time that she fell, she found a door that led into something that she didn't know but thought might be a jail – a dark cellar, a cave. At that point, she awakened with an unpleasant feeling. She then told me that every time she went to the city with the buildings that she had dreamed about, she passed by the monument-tomb. She then commented that it often happened that she would dream of falling and of having the sensation that something was swallowing her up. At other times, she dreamed of seeing a clock and of being anxious when she noticed that she was late by some hours in relation to the commitments she had. She felt like the White Rabbit in the story of Alice in Wonderland, who struggled and struggled and was always late.

I then told her that it seemed to me she was trying to talk about feelings that pertained to her body and her emotions, something that might have to do with her frequent visits to the hospital ever since she was little, which worried her and required her being able to think about and share.

She told me it didn't seem to her that things were like that. Ever since she was little, she hadn't remembered things – "I only remember that I went to the hospital willingly and then I went to McDonald's with my dad." She showed some surprise when she realized that even in the dream, she had gone there with her father.

After a moment in which she was absorbed in her thoughts, I pointed out to her that continuous falling could be related to the relapses of her illness; she appeared more ready to recognize the anxiety-provoking aspect of those experiences that seemed to imprison her in a dark place imbued with feelings of death, such as those that might be evoked by the image of a tomb.

We have already alluded to the fact that the close correlation between bodily experiences and mental development is a cornerstone of psychoanalytic thinking, starting from Freud (1923), who maintained that "the ego is first and foremost a bodily ego" (p. 26). Subsequently, the birth of the mind itself was conceived as an "imaginative elaboration of somatic parts, feelings, and functions" (Winnicott 1949, p. 244), and the body-mind issue became the crossroads of various theoretical elaborations and the intersection between different disciplines akin to psychoanalysis, such as the neurosciences.

The first acts of thinking are put together from movements and motoric patterns aimed at the maintenance of physiological balance, whose ruptures require a measure of work from the mind in order to overcome the frustrations that reality imposes on us, even if only in the form of intense physiological needs. The belief that experiences of the body and those of the mind belong to a substantially unified process in which the bodily register and the psychic one demonstrate deep and visceral correlations has not received adequate attention in the experience of illness when somatic processes express critical elements concomitantly with possible traumatic fault lines at a psychic level. The body in the hospital presents as an amalgamation of measurable functions and processes that can be evaluated; illness alters the balance of these processes and makes it necessary to restore their equilibrium.

Without lapsing into generalizations that fail to assign merit and evidence to the sensitivity of many persons and the many laudable exceptions, the hospital world is pervaded by a profound and deeply rooted division between body and mind: the *res extensa* and the *res cogitans* of Cartesian memory. In a legacy from the platonic tradition and the subsequent Christian tradition, body and soul are often viewed as opposite poles of a radical dualism.

On the other hand, the attempt on the part of the exact sciences to keep together the body experienced by the subject – that which phenomenology defines as *Leib*, "the body that I am" and the *Korper*, "the body that I have" – often ends up leading to an interventionist tendency that reduces the body to a summation of organs in which the *Korper* is imposed on the *Leib*.

As may have already been observed, in this personal journey of mine "from psychoanalysis to pediatrics" I have felt very close to some psychoanalysts who have studied in depth the relationships between psyche and soma – first of all, Winnicott and Bion. The works of Eugenio Gaddini have also been a constant source of reference over the course of my professional history; his entire article "Notes on the Mind-Body Question" (1987) has for me represented a sort of companion along the way. It was as though at each new reading, Gaddini offered new observations, as my experiences coalesced and were strengthened, little by little, allowing me to appreciate various deeper levels.

Another important contribution came from those who have studied the structure of health care organizations and the levels of communication and thinking that underlie them and who bring up for consideration the institutional culture, primarily founded on individuals' need to protect themselves from the suffering that an encounter with illness provokes in those who come into contact with it (Elliott Jaques, Isabel Menzies Lyth, José Bleger, Wilfred Bion, and in Italy, Francesco Corrao, Claudio Neri, Anna Ferruta, and Antonello Correale). I noticed that when it came time to begin thinking about writing a new contribution, the foregoing psychoanalytic contributors formed the theoretical base to which I returned and that always offered me new suggestions.

The mind and the body were two entities that I had to work to keep separate when my training led me to deepen the psychoanalytic experience and its rootedness in primary bodily sensations, while my professional practice in the hospital put me in contact with situations in which the body assumed a role in the foreground. And they were two entities that I had to work just as hard to keep together between the activity of the psychoanalyst in my office and that of a psychologist in the hospital. The medical sciences are often attentive to the importance that psychic organization plays in somatic organization, but this attention is essentially theoretical – almost an intellectual curiosity that is frequently discarded when attention to organic aspects prevails in those situations in which a mental component appears evident.

The medical culture and the psychoanalytic culture are both, in some ways, jealously possessive of their own scientific-cultural arenas and of their own interventional tools: they enjoy reciprocal respect as long as "each keeps to its own." But how does one distinguish the respective areas of intervention when faced with a new-born who has been in an incubator for a few days? Their vital functions are controlled by a monitor that closely watches blood saturation, cardiac rhythm, and other physiological parameters. Suddenly, the child is filled with extreme tension, extends his limbs, and cries – signs that make one think of the somatic, protomental component of Winnicott's "primitive anxieties" (1960, p. 588) or of the "nameless dread" described by Bion (1962, p. 96).

The child's suddenly altered parameters and crying demand the attention of the staff and the mother. The latter, with the delicacy and tenderness allowed by the cumbersome equipment that envelops her son, lets him feel her presence with hand contact that seems to breach the depth of the little one's sensitivity. It is a limited contact but an effective one, and slowly the crying dissipates, the bodily reactions diminish, and the various indices restabilize. The child's lungs, heart, and even his neuroendocrine system again reach a state of equilibrium. In situations like this one, I found myself thinking about the adult's capacity to tranquilize the child through treatments, thus containing his anxieties – what we might experience in caressing a frightened puppy.

Problems are hidden because an understanding of what is going on in such situations requires a double perspective of observation – psychic and somatic – like an object that in order to be observed in its various facets would require a double source of illumination, whereas the presence of only one light source would naturally leave out areas of shadow and obscurity. As long as there continue to be (at least) two light sources in this field, privileging one of them and its perspective, there is a risk of increasing the contrast with the shadowy zone, with the foreign nature of the mind that is expressed through the body or with the foreign nature of the body that takes shape in the mind.

Eugenio Gaddini's (1987) words masterfully describe the process of continuing convergences and divergences that characterize the rapport between medicine and psychoanalysis:

> For psychoanalysis, the body and mind form a functional "continuum," the main element of which is a process of differentiation going from body to mind, but through which psychoanalysis, going by way of the mind, can ultimately arrive at the body.
>
> [p. 315]

The relationship between medicine and psychoanalysis is complex, and the pathways between the two disciplines have been closely interwoven since the beginning. The life of Sigmund Freud itself tells us of the difficulties encountered in the relationship between psychoanalysis and health care institutions, from the beginning. If Freud's medical/biological training constituted the starting point of psychoanalytic thinking and clinical work, very quickly, the object of psychoanalytic study shifted to the individual's psychic experience and mental suffering, more than onto the body and physical illness.

Even though Freud, by overcoming great obstacles and difficulties in 1902, succeeded in obtaining the qualification of *privatdozent* at the University of Vienna – something that allowed him to continue a series of studies that made use of notable successes – he came to be designated "ordinary professor" only in 1920, and once his private profession began to take shape, he was not permitted to become a member of the faculty, and entrusted charitable duties were not assigned to him (Jones 1953). There still seemed to be a sort of attraction-repulsion on the part of medicine toward psychoanalysis. In a certain sense, psychoanalysis represented, in the eyes of the medical establishment, something that could be organized and incorporated only with difficulty, given its "strange" therapeutic method, somewhat lacking in protocols and guidelines.

The fact that psychoanalysis attends to the individual's needs interferes with an epistemological system that claims to base itself on the requirement of the actual objectivization of the exact sciences.

Medicine's model of intervention is based on the explicit manifestation of illness, for which it is necessary to concern oneself with the body as an organism. Referring to the patient's individuality, investigating the world of his affects and connections, has become a sort of luxury. When, however, the patient's emotional and social reality stand out as an integral part of his illness, the need to have contact with professionals who are interested in emotional dynamics in order to care for those aspects as well becomes almost "a necessary annoyance" – especially if the patient's individuality – or that of his family – has to struggle to keep within established rules and is seen as "creating problems."

Along this journey of attraction-repulsion, approaching-distancing, psychoanalysis runs the risk of losing its own specificity, becoming re-absorbed by disciplines that are more solidly located in the academic tradition, those that aspire to the usage of theoretical terms and constructs. In running the risk of making up their own and utilizing them beyond the theoretical context to which they refer, they lose their efficiency. In this case, psychoanalysis might become an *explanation* of a more pathological event, without the possibility of being actually applied.

An alternative is to propose the active involvement of caregivers in a new way of seeing things that presupposes at least a partial sharing of clinical practice and training methods, in which the psychological experience of clinical personnel will be an integrated part – not only that of the patient. My professional practice in the hospital has been characterized by a continual oscillation between these two alternatives.

Some Personal History

I have found myself working in this setting due to the coming together of some elements almost by chance. My motivations and my personal history have together formed a fertile ground for the realization of a productive experience.

One day, in my office that provided services to children in the area, where I had worked for almost 20 years in the realm of children's mental health, I got a phone call from a colleague who was leaving the hospital. She asked if I might be interested in taking over her position in the paediatric ward because she would like to leave it in the hands of someone who was in tune with her way of working. At first I was surprised, almost detached from the idea. I was halfway through my training with the Italian Psychoanalytic Society, still in analysis and in supervision to complete my credentials as a psychoanalyst. My relationship with public institutions had by now reached a terminus; I intended to dedicate myself exclusively to private practice.

I felt the weight of all the years of energy expended in interminable discussions between psychologists and neuropsychiatrists, between those of little knowledge and the more-or-less powerful entities, with conflicts among outpatient clinics, districts, quarters, and the various sectors of responsibility and working units of service. But the idea of starting to become part of an extensive hospital structure made me curious. "I'll try it," I told myself, and due to a series of favourable circumstances, after all the necessary administrative perambulations, at the beginning of the 2000s I began to work in the Department of Pediatrics in the Sant'Orsola-Malpighi University Hospital in Bologna.

I had in mind the work of colleagues in other settings – especially in France, where very rich experiences had been developed in institutional contexts. In particular, Didier Anzieu maintained that:

> Work of a psychoanalytic type must be done where the unconscious emerges. Standing, seated, or lying down – individually, in a group, or with the family – during the session, on the threshold of the door, at a hospital bedside, wherever a subject may be capable of showing his own anxieties and his own fantasies to someone who is supposed to be listening and is suited to giving explanations.
>
> [Anzieu 1975, p. 136]

Even though in the psychoanalytic field a great debate is presently opening up about extension of the method (Kaës 2015), for an analyst to work in a health care institution represents a risky game; in dealing with the area of early childhood, adolescence, and organic pathology, I have found myself having to resort to continual adjustments of technique in the attempt to response to the needs that have been presented little by little.

The doubt that has accompanied me in these attempts has been that of possibly lacking a fundamental core and the original identity of psychoanalysis or of falling into psychotherapeutic tendencies that could involve a structural modification of the technical mandate of psychoanalysis. This is not a new problem, and it is true that at the 1918 Congress in Budapest, Freud dedicated his paper to the problem of extending psychoanalysis to a broader sector of the population, asking himself whether "the large-scale application of our therapy will compel us to alloy the pure gold of analysis freely with the copper of direct suggestion"; rather, it was his hope that "whatever form this psychotherapy for the people may take, whatever the elements out of which it is compounded, its most effective and most important ingredients will assuredly remain those borrowed from strict and untendentious psycho-analysis" (Freud 1919, p. 168).

A psychoanalyst's work within a health care framework takes place, in fact, at the border of various often invisible frontier lines: between body and mind, between different medical specialties, between psychoanalysis and other forms of psychological intervention more focused on proscriptive aspects – rational, cognitive, or behavioural ones.

When I began to work in the hospital, it seemed to me I was led back to golden analytic currency to be spent in clinical work – coins that I had put aside over long years of analysis and training but that, notwithstanding the fact that they seemed extremely useful in situations that I found myself having to cope with, didn't seem to be the currency in use in the "hospital" territory. Expecting that the conditions would be created in which this currency could be used, I went around with these coins in my pocket, exchanging one now and then for a coin that purists would define as the up-to-date, bronze currency. Furthermore, if it is true that gold is always a sheltered asset that remains constant despite the financial volatility of the moment, at times, in going around with gold coins in one's pocket in the era of credit cards, virtual coins, and online banking, one risks being limited to the restricted niche of a collector.

As much as I had faith in my internal setting, in the analytic work of my private practice, and in meeting with my colleagues at various psychoanalytic institutions, I often asked myself whether, in the end, the psychological interventions in use in the hospital – which ranged from the normal basics of common sense and more or less behavioural forms of technique to correct and at times sophisticated interventions – didn't subsume all my resources, and in the end, perhaps little remained of the "analytic gold."

To keep these thoughts at bay, I preserved as indispensable my dedication to a certain number of hours of private practice in the analysis of adults, children, and adolescents, in order to maintain contact with deeper dimensions of transference – that is, to take account of the passage of unconscious elements between patient and analyst within the treatment relationship. At the same time, I dedicated my early years of practice to creating a space – physical, emotional, relational – that made it possible for me to know myself, as a person and as a professional – to know the possibilities, that is, of an occupation that took account of deeper factors than a superficial psychology of common sense.

Psychology and psychoanalysis – which common sense sees as one of its many variations – are often considered a sort of "parsley" – good for all kinds of soup, highly idealized when they are missing yet firmly devalued when brought forward – an oscillation, that is, between an idealizing emotional emphasis in every somatic manifestation and the complementary devaluation by which, in the end, one is seen to be able to do quite well while barely taking into account emotional experiences.

To demonstrate how little psychological aspects came to be considered in the hospital, after the person who had preceded me in this role had retired, his office disappeared, absorbed into the premises of another health care service, and my first years of work were carried out in completely unsuitable areas. In facing work conditions that at some moments were decisively disheartening, I found it useful to return to the memory of an anecdote that an analyst, Alfredo Spadoni, had related in a training seminar. It was about a French colleague who lived and worked in a modest house and who, every morning, carefully re-made the bed in which he had slept – which would then become the couch for his patients. "They don't come for the office, they come for you," Dr Spadoni declared.

Turning to past episodes of this type – to the people who taught us that the internal work setting and its characteristics are the basic ingredients of an intervention that wants to truly enter into contact with patients and promote developed relationships – has been the main impetus to go forward, to believe in what we are doing even at times in which, with patients waiting outside the door, we are forced to "re-make the bed" in a room pressed into a different service at night, outside the regular cleaning arrangement for official outpatient clinics.

I began to work. I became "the new psychologist" who tried to provide answers to various problems as they were presented, often charged with expectations as urgent and unrealistic as they were implicitly discrediting. There was a need for the previously mentioned "psychological parsley" – good for all soups but never missed if it was left out.

To follow on with a culinary metaphor dear to Antonino Ferro (1996), I tried to respond to the request for quick and economical foods in the psychological fast food business, leaving it to be intuited that the kitchen could provide something better and different as well. My basic ingredient in the kitchen consisted of recognizing that unconscious reality influences every human behaviour. I had faith in the ability to listen and an absolute awareness that some change is possible only through a modification of a person's internal configuration and not through instructions, advice, or psychological directives. Knowledge of the limits of our interventions and the refusal of a delegated task focusing on the oscillation between omnipotence and impotence were also ingredients used in all preparations, even in the most basic sauces.

Winnicott refers to the always indefinable novelty of the unconscious by referring to a poem from the Indian poet Tagore; he quotes Tagore as follows: "On the seashore of endless worlds, children play" (Winnicott 1971, p. 96). The idea of an area that may be at an intermediate level between the beach and the sea, between consciousness and the unconscious, where it is possible for there to be a space for personal developments and ever-changing expressions of psychic movements, has always fascinated me.

In hospital work, one is out on the open sea. The surface is always different; it can be calm (rarely) and flat or more often rippled by light breezes and at times lashed by stormy winds that interfere with navigation or risk creating the shipwrecks that one encounters in traveling. The ocean's depth, too, varies from a few centimetres to a great abyss.

The psychoanalyst in these situations, more interested in early experiences in the internal world than in more superficial external manifestations, operates with the methodical movements of a diver who owes to his respect for rules and technique the very possibility of staying alive, exploring the ocean floor at considerable depth. On the other hand, from a psychological point of view, in the hospital the activity looks more like that of a surfer who, thanks to a learned technique, is able to straddle the waves and arrive at the shoreline, at any rate, by entrusting himself to a different method.

Even the application of time is different. The methodical application of rules and schedules that contributes to the mixture of internal and external conditions underlying psychoanalytic intervention, also known as the setting, runs up against almost insurmountable difficulty. In the morning, one is ready with one's own surfboard to await the wave that, if everything goes well, will lead to our once again finding ourselves on the beach at the end of a day of work. At any rate, one must be able to stay on the surfboard; from there depths can be seen that will require future immersions, and one will pass close to the emerging rocks and the hidden rocks, knowing that ruptures will be experienced in which navigating with confidence is essential.

Inside the murkiness created by a complex hospital setting in which, within the work setting – with its precise hierarchical and cultural connotations – work groups come together, bonded by a feeling of resonance, over time acquaintance and reciprocal closeness are created with medical colleagues, perhaps at a more personal level than an institutional one. With some colleagues, I could share new experiences, curiosity, and tolerance for reciprocal differences; with others, I experienced a very meaningful collaboration; with still others, there was a polite distancing.

Over time, a group of young, very gifted psychology colleagues gradually formed around me, colleagues who had begun to work in specific areas, reaching a level of in-depth knowledge in their own spheres of intervention and at the same time starting out on individual training journeys in the psychodynamic and psychoanalytic field. Often placed beyond structured commitments and the assumption of responsibility on the part of corporate control, with private contributions and those from associations and at the initiative of various responsible parties, they created collaborations with psychologists who worked in the various settings, trying to fill a void in contact with patients whom the first to notice had been the caregiving doctors.

However, these were initiatives similar to "a leopard's spots," with a random distribution that could be defined as karstic or like porous limestone. One hoped that in the future some courageous administrator would induce a leap forward in quality, such that the big hospital structures would provide organizational placements for psychology, as well as systematic endowments that would insert it – with full legitimacy and with maximal possibilities for intervention – into the complex machine of health care firms.

The metaphor of the foreign body – which has been used, as mentioned, since the beginning of psychoanalytic history to illustrate defensive processes mobilized by the psychic apparatus to cope with traumatic experience – is often re-presented in the course of my work. I myself have experienced the feeling of being a foreign body in a culture in which reflective thinking aimed at the search for psychic truth often assumes the character of an irritating thorn. And I felt myself to be a foreign body when my professional approach aroused defensive reactions or when I noticed a gap between the potential linked to psychoanalytic culture and practice and other psychological techniques, essentially psychotherapeutic ones.

At the same time, my membership in a member society of the International Psychoanalytical Association (IPA) signified, for me, feeling the responsibility of being part of an ancient tradition, proven on the clinical level and having solid scientific bases, one that allowed me to be trained in very rigorous didactic institutions.[1]

The impression is that often in the medical world and in the external world in general, in consequence of substantial neglect of psychoanalysis, the added value of training and preparation according to particularly rigorous criteria is not at all appreciated. If such experiences are useful to a psychologist or a psychiatrist, their training and technical orientations often assume only marginal importance.

Regarding clinical applications of psychoanalysis in medicine as well, one nonetheless observes an alternation of periodic moments of contact and distancing by which much psychoanalytic knowledge has entered the medical world. In fact, psychoanalytic models are referred to frequently in clinical work, often as an added explanation or, in cases of considerable uncertainty, utilizing the concepts of the unconscious, the internal world, childhood sexuality, and transference.

Psychoanalysis has progressed by developing its theory and technique around the analyst-patient relationship. The psychoanalytic exercise requires a long and complex journey in which elements of a professional nature are intertwined with the psychoanalyst's personal development. The acquisition of a stable analytic function that can manage contact with patients' deepest areas in therapeutic relationships requires that theoretical contents learned during training be rooted in personal experience in the working through of the future analyst's deep areas of personal human experience.

I think that an important factor in overcoming many conflictual situations may be represented by my ongoing presence, just as I maintain that the presence in health care institutions of psychoanalysts – who can give live testimony of a culture and a specific way of reading problems and confronting them – constitutes an important promotional tool for psychoanalysis outside its traditional borders (outreach).

I consider it very positive, for example, that some candidates and members of the psychoanalytic society are part of the contracted hospital staff, just as many who are specializing in legitimate schools of psychoanalytic psychotherapy have identified the hospital as a place for their practical training. In addition, it seems to me of no small importance that, thanks to the presence of psychoanalysis in places to which requests for intervention are addressed, the majority of patients can turn to colleagues with a specific area of competence. Among many persons, it is thought appropriate that because a psychoanalyst can fulfil a function of cultural transformation within a health care institution, it is necessary that his presence enjoy a sufficient level of stability and that he can count on a working relationship of a minimum duration of time (see Carbone 2003, 2009).

One cannot help but agree with Roussillon (1988), who supports the importance of the presence of the psychoanalyst in health care institutions, emphasizing that

> the expert must have enough times when he is present in the institution, and on the other hand, he must have managed to carve out a recognized territory for himself in the institution – that his personal qualities and practical attitude have given him the idea of a "container" that is sufficiently good and trustworthy, and ultimately that one doesn't find oneself in an overly hierarchical position nor involved in power struggles.

[p. 201]

Without a position in the field that transforms the disturbing presence of psychoanalytic thinking into a possible therapeutic option and into a working tool to which one can turn, the risk is that psychoanalysis itself will become a foreign body and that the organism's reactions will be mobilized toward it – an irritating process that forms the basis for an expulsion. Psychoanalysis, from an organizational business point of view, becomes a fragmented vessel in the middle of other specialties that have solid academic and organizational traditions – a young science that cannot count on established structures and hierarchies, one that introduces a disturbing element in environments that are not very disposed toward uncertainty or doubt, waiting for conditions to be created for its expulsion. Once outside the system, it is not easy to resist the pipe dreams provided by more superficial techniques that don't allow for much discussion of professional or institutional equilibrium.

In Plain Language

Within the limits of possibility, in writing this book, I have tried to give a voice to a request that patients make of those who take care of them. "Doctor, say it to me in plain language" has often been said to me in conversations with persons to whom their condition had been described in exemplary but incomprehensible scientific terms. In working in a border area, I felt the duty of making my thinking comprehensible and making my words simple. It is an effort that aims at simplifying the language that we often use in our meetings and that at times ends up being incomprehensible, even to people with advanced learning in other fields of knowledge.

I can confirm that this tendency toward simplification is a struggle that pays off; we cannot overestimate how much unconscious defences – which are there and are very active – contribute to intolerance for a language that can be comprehended only with difficulty and that often characterizes our technical jargon. I tried to use the experience of persons whom I considered my teachers – those who spoke of complex arguments while using a language that even a child would have understood. First among these was Marcella Balconi.

In this book, aimed at those not trained in a professional specialty, some of the contributions that "the foreign body" of psychoanalysis can bring into the field of health care are proposed. There are illustrations of the conceptual contribution of psychoanalysis, with its listening theories – on trauma, on therapeutic factors, on psychic pain – in order to understand the clinical conditions in which there is a predominantly emotional aetiology.

In the main part, there are illustrations of the various forms of psychotherapy that draw on psychoanalysis: individual psychotherapy, parent-child psychotherapy, group psychotherapy, and various formats according to the needs of the persons involved and the characteristics of various charitable contexts.

And finally, the activity of workers with psychodynamic training is taken into consideration – training in promoting and conducting work groups to encourage the reading of emotional aspects in various institutional settings, reflecting on the role of discussion groups and supervision in clinical activities.

Note

1 The psychoanalyst's training is acquired through a program that requires the trainee to subject himself to a personal analysis in order to gain maximal awareness of his own areas of suffering and conflict, necessary for bringing a therapeutic vocation to fruition – a necessity that, if not adequately dealt with, could interfere with the analyst's work with patients. Beyond a personal analysis and theoretical seminars, in order to attain the qualification of psychoanalyst, it is necessary to conduct supervised therapies within a training program that requires on average about ten years. What characterizes the clinical practices of psychoanalysts and differentiates them from various other therapists who draw on psychoanalytic discourse at an intellectual level is that the conducting of clinical experiences presupposes continuous work with oneself and with colleagues in a process of ongoing training in which personal and professional aspects evolve in well-constructed encounters with a community of colleagues at local, national, and international levels.

References

Anzieu, D. (1975). La psychanalyse encore. *Revue française de psychanalyse*, 39(1–2): 135–146.

Bion, W. R. (1962). *Learning from Experience*. Lanham, MD: Jason Aronson/Rowman & Littlefield, 2004.

Breuer, J. & Freud, S. (1893). On the psychical mechanism of hysterical phenomena: Preliminary communication. *S. E.*, 2.

Carbone, P. (2003). *Le ali di Icaro: rischio e incidenti in adolescenza [The Wings of Icarus: Risk and Accidents in Adolescence]*. Torino: Bollati Boringhieri.

———. (2009). Adolescenti, medici e malattie. Una psicoanalista in corsia [Adolescents, doctors and illnesses: A psychoanalyst on the hospital ward]. In *Essere Adolescenti Oggi [Being an Adolescent Today]*, ed. R. Goisis & S. Bonfiglio. Milano: I Quaderni del Centro Milanese di Psicoanalisi.

Ferro, A. (1996). *In the Analyst's Consulting Room*, trans. P. Slotkin. Hove, UK: Brunner-Routledge.

Freud, S. (1919). Lines of advance in psycho-analytic therapy. *S. E.*, 17.

———. (1923). The ego and the id. *S. E.*, 19.

Gaddini, E. (1987). Notes on the mind-body question. *Int. J. Psychoanal.*, 68:315–329.

Goisis, P. R. (2014). *Costruire l'adolescenza: tra immedesimazione e bisogni [Building Adolescence between Identifications and needs]*. Milano-Udine: Mimesis Edizioni.

Jones, E. (1953). *The Life and Work of Sigmund Freud*. New York: Basic Books, 1975.

Kaës, R. (2015). *Pour une métapsychologie de troisième type*. Paris: Dunot Editeur.

Laufer, E. (2005). The body as an internal object. *Adolescence*, 23(2):363–379.

Mancia, M. (2004). *Sentire le parole. Archivi sonori della memoria implicita e musicalità del transfert [Hearing the Words: The Auditory Archives of Implicit Memory and the Musicality of the Transference]*. Torino: Bollati Boringhieri, 2006.

Nicolò, A. M. (a cura di). (2009). *Adolescenza e violenza [Adolescence and Violence]*. Roma: Il Pensiero Scientifico Editore.

Racamier, P. C. (1970). *Le psychanalyste sans divan: la psychanalyse et les institutions de soins psychiatriques* (Vol. 24). Paris: Payot.

Riolo, F. (2009). Lo statuto psicoanalitico di inconscio. *Rivista di Psicoanalisi*, 55:11–28.

Roussillon, R. (1988). Spazi e pratiche istituzionali. Il ripostiglio e l'interstizio [Institutional spaces and practices: The cupboard and the crevice]. In *L'Istituzione e le istituzioni [The Institution and Institutions]*, ed. J. Bleger, E. Enriquez, R. Kaës, F. Fornari, P. Faustier, R. Roussillon & J. P. Vidal. Roma: Borla, 1991.

Ruggiero, I. (2016). Il corpo ripudiato. In *La mente adolescente e il corpo ripudiato [The Adolescent Mind and the Repudiated Body]*, ed. A. M. Nicolò & I. Ruggiero. Milano: FrancoAngeli.

Winnicott, D. W. (1949). Mind and its relation to the psyche-soma. In *From Paediatrics to Psychoanalysis*. New York: Brunner-Routledge, 1992, pp. 243–254.

———. (1960). The theory of the parent-infant relationship. *Int. J. Psychoanal.*, 41:585–595.

———. (1971). *Playing and Reality*. London: Tavistock Publications.

Chapter 1

The Basic Therapeutic Factor

It may seem strange for a book written by a psychoanalyst to begin by stating that in health care facilities, psychology is not exclusive to psychologists or to other professionals who have a "psy-" prefix in their qualifications or job title.

Notwithstanding the particular attributes of psychoanalysis and its clinical applications and the specific expertise of different health care clinicians, there are nonspecific therapeutic elements in their common heritage. These therapeutic elements characterize every health care intervention for another human being that is intended take care of his needs. These elements are also alive in paediatrics.

That is to say, the idea of psychology as the exclusive province of the "psy-" professional reflects a lack of integration of the various types of knowledge and interventions. The idea of separating the emotional care from somatic interventions or outsourcing it to side professionals could obstruct the development of the vision of the patient as a whole.

Children in the Hospital

Children encounter the hospital for an endless array of issues – for health problems that are congenital, chronic, acute, benign, and sometimes more serious, in some cases even lethal. In all these situations, the principal task that little patients and their parents find themselves faced with is that of identifying a meaning, both in experiences and in the body – or, to start from the body, in what they come to experience in the encounter with the hospital. It is essential to be able to speak of these things and to think about them in a way that gives them a name and that allows a sharing of the sensations and emotions stimulated by them. If I had to express in concise terms the main psychological function of a health care worker in the hospital context, I would say that, beyond treatment and cure, it is the capacity to listen and to seek the meaning of the various situations in which it falls to him to intervene – and to propose a culture of bonding in place of a culture of avoidance, spitting, and fragmentation.

Meaning and truth, connections and ties that permit the bringing together of energy with representations and allow one to give a shape to phantasms, are contrasted with the experience of anxiety. The appearance of feelings, words, and

DOI: 10.4324/9781003252238-2

mental representations allows traumatic experiences, too, to become assimilated. These representations are difficult to access at the level of mental representation because they are too intense, or they are limited to something that took place at a physical/sensorial level and has not reached the possibility of being transformed into material accessible by the psychic apparatus.

Almost every day I have found myself agreeing with Bion (1965) that healthy mental development depends on truth, just as a living organism depends on food.[1] This is true both in individual terms and in institutional group functioning; it is a *nonspecific* therapeutic factor, the minimum basic element for a meaningful encounter with the other. Or, to state it more accurately, it is a *specific* therapeutic factor common to the various professions that address treatment (Berti Ceroni 2005) – doctors, nurses, technical personnel, and (why not?) administrators, given the ever greater impact that administrative personnel have on people who make use of health care services.

The acquisition of this therapeutic factor lies outside various technical and specialized skills and is based on reflection on one's own professional activity. It requires basic personal endowments and is achieved through implicit learning that often occurs almost by osmosis, from contact with colleagues who adopt a professional style that inspires it. Rarely in updated professional practices or in training initiatives is adequate importance attributed to this type of culture, in contrast to the attention given to technical proficiency that has been firmly established and can be codified.

Yet this is something that psychoanalytic culture has situated at the foundation of clinical practice: the capacity to listen and to be in contact with another's suffering, with one's own, and with the way in which, through the encounter, the one resonates with the other. In other words, what Reik (1948) defined as "the third ear": the capacity to be attuned to another's emotional states and, at the same, to one's own. The listening to which psychoanalysis refers aims at the possibility of attending to hidden emotions in the encounter with the other and of establishing an attunement with what the other is expressing beyond the format or words that are used on the surface.

According to Reik, the third ear constitutes a sense organ that joins with the other five senses and can promote better listening not only to what takes place in the patient but also and especially to what is taking place in the therapist. Mario Rossi Monti (2006) emphasizes a dual function as uniquely characteristic of the third ear, which according to Reik must not be confused with an internal ear.

> In fact, on the one hand, the third ear "captures" what the other person hears or thinks, but does not reach the point of expressing it in words. But on the other hand, beyond being directed toward the imperceptible and minimal signs that are necessarily mostly dispersed, the third ear must be turned toward what is inside the analyst – to hear voices from the internal part of the self that would otherwise end up drowned by the noise of the knowing processes of thinking.
> [Rossi Monti 2006, translation by G. Atkinson]

Attention to the meaning expressed through a condition of illness or discomfort in a listening dimension constitutes the emotional background that, whether specifically intended or not, to a greater or lesser degree, forms the basis of every intervention directed for another human being, whether child or adult. Such an intervention recognizes the patient as having his own point of view on things and the competence to decide to attend to his own improvement.

A medical colleague introduces me to Alessandra and her mother, Francesca. Alessandra is fourteen years old, and for more than five years, she and her mother have travelled throughout the country in search of an organic cause for a continual contracture of her calf muscle, which not even the latest cerebral and peripheral MRI's have managed to reveal. Now her parents don't know how to react when Alessandra calls them and asks that they pick her up at school because her leg is bothering her; she experiences their attempts to convince her to stick it out as a lack of interest in her.

In my first meeting with the parents, the possibility emerges that emotional factors are playing a role in Alessandra's symptomatology. Her grandparents and the family of her mother's sister live near her home, and it has long been their habit to come to the home of Alessandra and her parents for lunches and dinners, where everyone eats together. This custom arose spontaneously when Alessandra's mother, Francesca, had begun to cook for her own parents and for her sister and her family. At these meals, Alessandra had for a long time been the centre of everyone's attention – including that of her aunt's husband, who in the meantime had reunited with his own nuclear family – until Alessandra reached the age of seven, when a little cousin was born. This cousin attracted all the adults' attention – and apparently Alessandra's as well, as she seemed to want to take care of him. According to her mother, "there's a bit of a mixed blessing" since Alessandra has always been a calm child, while the new arrival is somewhat "overbearing."

It is hard for Alessandra and her parents to find moments to be alone, and accepting the situation of a big, undifferentiated family has not been easy either for Francesca or for Alessandra, who hasn't managed to distinguish herself from her family as a daughter. Her mother maintains that this is a problem she herself has had, though she is nearly 50 years old: "At a personal level, I overcame it, I sealed it up" – even though she believes that this situation may in part have been responsible for a past difficulty that led her to consult a psychologist about a problem of being overweight.

"Since this has been a problem for me, I didn't want it to be one for Alessandra," says her mother, who in all these years has not been able to assign a mental meaning to her daughter's malaise. She identifies as her daughter's problem – beyond the loss of her role in the family – the fact that the little cousin has become an "invading presence" to whom Alessandra often reacts by closeting herself in her room. As she says these things, Francesca remembers having herself been jealous of her little sister.

At the end of this first session, I imagine the big dinner table around which an expanded family consumes lunch and dinner, leaning on Alessandra's mother, who hasn't managed to differentiate herself from her nuclear family and who now sees her own suffering expressed in the tension in her daughter's leg. On a symbolic level, this leg tension seems to indicate a struggle to bear the weight of the situation.

The parents gladly acquiesce to my proposal of working with them, and Alessandra does, too, although she imposes a condition: that of speaking only with me, making clear from the beginning her need to have a separate space that supports her project of individuating herself as an autonomous subject.

Alessandra tells me at the first session that now her leg pains her a little less but that when it is bad, "it makes me cry – the pain is unbearable – even pain pills are less effective now." She hopes that "this thing," our work together, will attenuate the problem somewhat, that I will help her unblock herself, help her overcome the feeling of not being understood even when it happens that she has a fight with her little cousin.

> Until the age of seven, I was 'waited on and revered'; then my cousin arrived and upset my life somewhat. He took away the attention that I got earlier. I feel cast aside; the more he grows, the more he takes up space.

She does not completely mind the expanded family – which, however, in her opinion, also has many disadvantages. She speaks of her attempts to be more autonomous and to go out alone but complains that her parents are "afraid of the black man." She herself is more adaptable, she says, and then intends to tell me that, if her parents set limits "it's not a Greek tragedy," but she makes a slip and instead says, "it's not a Greek wrestling match." She is subsequently able to accept my observation that her metaphor is more appropriate to a type of struggle or fight than it is to an adaptation.

At our second meeting, Alessandra says that things are going somewhat better, and her leg hasn't hurt her during this period. She doesn't know why not – whether it's because she has changed or her relationship with her parents has changed.

I talk to her about a leg that seemed to be struggling to keep its footing in a difficult situation, but now that someone has noticed the fact that, through the leg, she has been trying to make it understood that something isn't going well, it can relax. "What do you think the leg is saying now?" I ask her. She says, "Now it's not saying anything."

She expresses feeling extremely moved when she talks about herself, about her plan to leave home and live alone at age 18. When I speak to her about the fact that I can share her desire for her own space without fear of being bad or of causing harm to anyone, she answers: "I would like them to understand my point of view, my need to detach myself." She thinks that her parents, too, are in some way living her situation, even though they travelled a great deal to try to help with her leg before reaching the understanding that this was something else: the desire to walk her own path, to conclude a journey of adolescent separation, with all the grieving connected to that, to unblock Alessandra in the process of subjectivization.[2]

Emotional Factors and Professional Choices

In implicit fantasies about our professional choices, one can often find the belief that by curing others, we can repair missing elements and suffering that we notice signs of in ourselves. There is often an overvaluation of our capacities and skills; we think that there's a reason for everything, and that we can find an explanation. Indeed, we implicitly believe that the other's well-being depends on our capacity to find solutions, to illuminate areas of uncertainty. It is difficult to accept that the cure takes time, and it is not always possible to achieve.

In a culture very much driven toward *doing*, like that of medicine, which one must often confront when there are acute problems, paradoxically, the psychologist is often asked *not to do* – not to give answers or prescriptions, to be an interpreter of the "negative capability" that Bion cited: "when a man is capable of being in uncertainties, mysteries, doubts, without any irritable reaching after fact and reason" (Keats quoted by Bion 1970, p. 125 – *Attention and Interpretation*).

The way of approaching people is thus modified and tends to shift away from what Dina Vallino (2009) called "the consultation of dependence." As we will see later on in this book, the traditional therapist-patient relationship, in which there is someone who has information and someone else who receives it, can be reimagined as a "participatory consultation." In this model, the therapist functions almost in the background, aiming at the creation of conditions, the construction of coordinates according to which another person can find his own solutions, rescuing the thoughts being discussed from the presence of an excessive quantity of affects and sensations. If creating the conditions and the emotional space that foster thinking seem to be the principal characteristic of the psychological endeavour – a gift that many clinicians have refined into an individual sensitivity and a well-established experience – in the arenas in which I have worked, too, there are places in which these same processes take place.

Health care institutions are complex organizations in which the broadest levels of emotional exchange and the most diverse iterations of group life are interwoven. There are layers of technical institutional management, hierarchical professional roles and functions in the life of an institutions. These layers may be integrated to a greater or lesser extent, with the ideas at the foundation. In a paediatric hospital, these include the fight against illnesses and death that threaten children's existence and the risk of becoming immersed in unbearable pain in the parent-child relationship.

Sometimes organizations adopt systems of functioning that perpetuate levels of suffering in individuals, workers, or end users, as well as in work groups. Their very characteristics seem to derive from the need to defend those who belong to the group or those close to it, against mental pain by adopting mechanisms that avoid contact and the establishment of connections. In many instances such manoeuvres nearly serve to compound human suffering but in reality end up perpetuating the suffering.

More than 50 years ago, Isabel Menzies Lyth (1960), following the path initiated by Elliott Jaques (1955), emphasized the function of health care institutions as a system of protection against the primitive anxieties that patients' pathologies could evoke in health care personnel. She referred to the intensity and violence of the libidinal and aggressive fantasies that characterize a person's first moments of life and contribute to the constitution of a world populated by wounded and damaged internal objects. According her now classic paper that seems to have withstood the test of time (Lawlor 2009), she stressed the fact that contact with patients and their family members reactivates the internal reality of such intense and scarcely bearable fantasies, so that it is often necessary to activate the protective mechanisms that underlie the working methods and culture of therapeutic institutions.[3]

I came across Menzies's paper at the beginning of my professional career. The paper accompanied me over time as a recurrently constant presence. From time to time, I take up the paper to explore the ideas more deeply. Along my analytic and training journey as well, I was able to recognize and appreciate the degree to which our professional choices are born of the need to care for ourselves – for the parts of ourselves that we feel are immature, undervalued or irreparably damaged. We can come to the point of saying that the subsequent process of vocational maturation consists of a gradual coming to terms with these parts in a more realistic way, renouncing omnipotent fantasies and recognizing our limits and our therapeutic possibilities.

Health care organizations are implicitly structured according to criteria that guarantee the management of anxiety stemming from the encounter with broken lives and the borders between life and death – that in a hospital come in many guises, from when one launches on a procreative project to when an event of any type endangers an existence that is already underway. These ways of functioning have a certain professional transgenerational transmission stemming from a foundational myth (Kaës 1988). They are transmitted, that is, with the same style over the course of working generations. Today's directors retain the characteristics of their predecessors and only rarely succeed in transcending their personal formulations to the persons who work with them.

It may happen that in the same institutional environment, various departments have engraved at access portals – invisible to the eye but extremely pervasive in daily routines – the implicit rules of behaviour to which everyone clings in every eventuality, in order not to be exposed to isolation and individual suffering. These are indispensable survival methods that enable us to maintain contact with the suffering, pain, and death to which we are exposed. But these mechanisms also exact a high emotional price. These conditions could be negotiated if the complex experiences of the people who use them could find a means of expression – including emotional aspects – and if within the organization a path could also be cleared toward a way of listening to these dimensions (see the chapter on groups with the personal).

These are dimensions of professional experience and of expressions of a humanity that is too often constricted in the norms of institutional behaviour. Those elements, following subterranean pathways, vital sensations, and areas of creative functioning, continue to flow and to give meaning to the relationships between people.

Interstitial Spaces

Rousillon (1988) brought to light the function of what he defines as *interstitial spaces*, which Bolognini and Trombini (1994) identified, for example, in electrical hot plates that allow makeshift coffeepots to function – and today, perhaps, automatic dispensers in the little kitchenettes with which every department is endowed. This is the place where vital, human spaces most often find expression.

In effect, there are departments with a more developed psychological culture in which the responsible persons are aware that an important part of their role consists of fostering communication among work group members, that they are the trusted ones who organize activities, taking into account the group's growth and the fact that no professional should live in an individual dimension. In those departments, priority is given to relational aspects through staff meetings and briefings at regular intervals, sometimes daily. These are demanding experiences but very rewarding ones when we consider the quality of the department's work, experiences that frequently enter into a collision course with hierarchical organizational levels based on the evasion of anxiety, which cannot tolerate the act of sharing difficulties, affects, and types of knowledge (Correale 2006).

In the paediatric division of Sant'Orsola Hospital in Bologna, beyond kitchenettes and rare periods of training and professional updates that are also aimed at people's emotions, there is a place that belongs to everyone and that escapes rigid definition and conflicts transmitted to this or that structure or operative unity. It is a constantly well-maintained area, clean – a sort of "nobody's place" and at the same time one that belongs to everyone. It is a type of extraterritorial space in an environment in which subtle, invisible, powerful, and often fixed enclosures have always divided every space and every area of activity, according to criteria that are buried deep in the mists of time and that stubbornly resist every attempt at modification or integration.

I refer to the sculpture representing a Madonna and child located in the area in front of the paediatric hospital. It is a copy of a Madonna by Jacopo della Quercia that dominates the main entrance to Bologna's Basilica of San Petronio. It is a statue of great beauty representing a seated Madonna. With an absorbed air and an apparently detached gaze, she holds a child on her lap, a child who almost uses her as a stable base to lean upon, who seems to push himself out to the world and the life before him. The sculpture is a discrete presence that each person can come to when he most needs to, summer or winter, day or night, in a transitional but slightly secluded zone that is constantly enlivened by unseen hands that maintain it, continuously decorating it with fresh flowers or entrusting it with little votive objects.

It is unusual that, passing through here, there will not be someone who feels the sculpture's presence as an integrating part of hospital life and who doesn't at least direct a distracted greeting to the Madonna during the course of a day. And she is there, available to meet anyone who decides to stop even for a moment and to gather up whatever thoughts may be brought to her – almost as if, by her very existence, she expresses the possibility of giving shape to unthinkable ideas and projects, of an opportunity to consign all the hopes and fears that go beyond the possibility of thinking to a steady and trustworthy entity. She seems to listen, to allow people to express their most intense pain and their most secret hope.

She is placed in the open, in a position peripheral to the hospital's management centres and outside the walls of the scientific and technological parameters ruled by other divinities and their rituals. The paternal god of technomedicine of exact sciences, of the principles of technical objectives, has often already expressed commandments, has uttered words that the human mind is not always able to process and that can require time to be able to assimilate and transform into real awareness.

Undoubtedly, that little Madonna is the expression of a religious faith in which the Madonna is an integrating and fundamental component but also lies beyond a strictly religious vision. It seems to me that this sculptural pair – and the possibility that it seems to permit being freely used by whoever turns to it – together with the Madonna's gaze that appears dreamy, can make us think of the reverie function that Bion (1962) identified as the basis of the maternal function. It is a function that the child learns in the early phases of life through the unfolding of experiences connected to the physical and emotional exchange in which the mother is able to gather into herself the feelings that the baby directs to her, allowing the experience of refinding one's own private mental contents, now cleansed of the characteristics that had made them indigestible and something impossible to confront.

The self's acquisition of this function of mental elaboration of somatic sensations and early emotional contents consists in the child's conquest of the possibility of thinking – a skill that, even when acquired to a sufficient degree, is never actually definitively accomplished. It risks breaking down under the impact of events and life phases that are particularly critical or emotional or in the presence of other especially intense affects. States of illness, pain, and grief require a difficult task of mental integration that sometimes transcends the individual's psychic capabilities, especially when one enters the area of "trauma" that by definition consists of the eruption of a quantity of emotions and excitations that exceed the capacities of the psychic apparatus. For the parents of hospitalized children, turning to that image allows hope to be kept alive and psychic life not to be undone by pain.

The function of the Madonna statue at Sant'Orsola Hospital, like every work of art in which one finds much of the artist's experience, seems to refer to a function of basic mirroring and self-formation. Lacan (1949), in his study of the mirror stage, speaks of the child's experience when, on seeing his image in the mirror together with that of the mother who holds him in her arms, loses himself in a sensation of euphoria that goes on to set the tone of the underlying sense of self. It is a concept that was again taken up by Winnicott (1971); and we can imagine that the person who sees the Madonna and experiences with her an intimate feeling of emotional closeness may come into contact with the early phases of his own development, phases in which there was an environment surrounding the self that welcomed and sustained, in which security and integrity could be taken for granted.

Whether we are aware of it or not, people continually direct these kinds of feelings toward us, and we can welcome them and participate together with the patient in a process of transformation and personal growth, or we can refuse them, overlook their need to be held, separate ourselves with our technical expertise, enclosing ourselves within the correctness of our technical responses. That highlights the function of listening and acceptance that I maintain represents a characteristic of interpersonal relationships that is especially active in the remedial professions.

Elements of this type are at play when we live the experience of listening – when we hear that a parent is bringing us something that worries him and is not amenable to mental elaboration, and after a conversation, he goes away with a different mindset. We don't know precisely what we have done, but we might imagine that we have listened to his worries, and even with our having only taken it into our mind, his concerns may have had some of their disquieting elements filtered out.

One of the principal sources of misunderstanding in relationships with children's parents that can occur in the hospital is our considering them to be perfectly rational people with whom it is possible to have a relationship of the same type as the convivial one that we have with anyone whom we happen to meet in everyday life. Sometimes things can be like that, but often the relationship parents have with us is characterized by the need to find a solution to a problem that greatly disturbs them, and that is tied to the well-being of what they hold most dear – their children – and that may appear to be irreparably compromised. Behind the appearance of an encounter similar to many in everyday life, a relationship is played out in which a person in a fragile and needy state turns to someone whom he imagines has the solution to his problems and who therefore appears to be characterized by the possession of ideal traits. The words spoken in the many exchanges that a doctor or a psychologist has in the course of a day, for that specific person, represent definitive answers, engraved on the stone of suffering emotionality, which remain unaltered even over the course of years – a memory that does not fade.

The doctor-patient or therapist-patient relationship develops within a subtle game of expectations about the person and the institution to which he belongs, which cannot be taken for granted and which in this chapter I have set out to explore and deepen.

Notes

1   "Healthy mental growth seems to depend on truth as the living organism depends on food" (Bion 1965, p. 38 – *Transformations*).
2   For more about the process of subjectivization, see Cahn's (2009) elaboration.
3   They essentially consist of the following: splits in the worker-patient relationship, depersonalization, negation of the value of individuality, self-detachment and denial of feelings, the attempt to eliminate decisions by adhering to ritual duties, reducing the weight of responsibility inherent in decisions through verifications and counterverifications, carrying out a collusive redistribution of responsibilities and nonresponsibilities, deliberately sought nonclarity in the distribution of responsibilities and reduction of their impact through delegation to superior positions, idealizing or devaluing the possibilities of individual growth – and, last, opposing all change.

References

Berti Ceroni, G. B., ed. (2005). *Come cura la psicoanalisi? [How Does Psychoanalysis Cure?]* Milano: FrancoAngeli.
Bion, W. R. (1962). *Learning from Experience*. London: William Heinemann.
———. (1965). *Transformations*. London: William Heinemann.
———. (1970). *Attention and Interpretation*. London: Tavistock.
Bolognini, S. & Trombini, G. (1994). Due psicoanalisti riflettono su come logora curare [Two psychoanalysts reflect on how the cure wears out the caregiver]. In *Come logora curare, medici e psicologi sotto stress [How the Cure Wears Out the Caregiver: Doctors and Psychologists under Stress]*, ed. G. Trombini. Bologna: Zanichelli.
Cahn, R. (2009). Una vita di lavoro con gli adolescenti [A life working with adolescents]. In "Essere Adolescenti oggi" ["Being Adolescents Today"], ed. R. Goisis & S. Bonfiglio. *I quaderni del Centro Milanese di Psicoanalisi [Notes from the Milanese Psychoanalytic Center]*. Milano: Centro Milanese di Psicoanalisi Cesare Musatti.
Correale, A. (2006). *Area traumatica e campo istituzionale [The Traumatic Area and the Institutional Field]*. Roma: Borla.
Jaques, E. (1955). Social systems as a defense against persecutory and depressive anxiety. In *New Directions in Psycho-Analysis*, ed. M. Klein, P. Heimann & R. E. Money-Kyrle. London: Karnac.
Kaës, R. (1988). Realtà psichica e sofferenza nelle istituzioni [Psychic reality and suffering in institutions]. In *L'istituzione e le istituzioni [The Institution and the Institutions]*, ed. J. Bleger, E. Enriquez, R. Kaës, F. Fornari, P. Faustier, R. Roussillon & J. P. Vidal. Roma: Borla, 1991.
Lacan, J. (1949). The mirror stage as formative of the *I* function. In *Écrits*, trans. B. Fink. New York/London: W. W. Norton, 2006.
Lawlor, D. (2009). Test of time: A case study in the functioning of social systems as a defence against anxiety: Rereading 50 years on. *Clin. Child Psychology & Psychiatry*, 14:523–530.
Menzies Lyth, I. (1960). A case-study in the functioning of social systems as a defence against anxiety. *Hum. Relat.*, 13(2):95–121.
Reik, T. (1948). *Listening with the Third Ear*. Boston, MA: Colonial Press.
Rossi Monti, M. (2006). *Paula Heimann: controtransfert e dintorni [Countertransference and Its Surroundings]*. Paper presented at Bologna Psychoanalytic Center.

Rousillon, R. (1988). Spazi e pratiche istituzionali. Il ripostiglio e l'interstizio [Institutional spaces and practices: The storeroom and the interstices]. In *L'istituzione e le istituzioni [The Institution and the Institutions]*, ed. J. Bleger, E. Enriquez, R. Kaes, F. Fornari, P. Faustier, R. Roussillon & J. P. Vidal. Roma: Borla, 1991.

Vallino, D. (2009). *Fare psicoanalisi con genitori e bambini [Doing Psychoanalysis with Parents and Children]*. Roma: Borla.

Winnicott, D. W. (1971). *Playing and Reality*. London: Routledge, 2005.

Chapter 2

Neonates, Pain, and Memory

In observing children and infants – even very young ones – who are faced with mental or physical suffering, one asks oneself what recollection they will be able to have of those early painful events. In those situations, it can also happen that one will hear remarks of a type suggesting that "crying makes one's eyes beautiful" and "crying strengthens the lungs," or one may hear it said that little children do not remember or that they recall only a little of what happens to them at a tender age.

In this chapter, we will consider whether and in what way early experiences can be transformed into solidified feelings fixed into the memory, influencing the child's mental development and maintaining that influence on adult life. The issue is not a simple one because it must be located at the very origin of psychic life, in time and personal space, in a complex area of transition between the body and the mind: where mental activity emerges from its physiological underpinnings.

Traditionally, psychoanalysis has been interested in ideational contents connected to unconscious activities that – exposed to the work of repression, through transformative processes – reach the point of expressing themselves in mental representations, in images, figures, words. Over time, especially with the work of Melanie Klein and the post-Kleinian development, importance has been assigned to the development of early fantasies connected to the initial stages of the child's life, which organize psychic life and maintain their influence over the course of his existence.

Thus, analysis finds itself confronting not only the recovery of repressed memories but also the completion of psychic acts not previously accomplished and hence "unformulated" – that is, not translated into thoughts. They are representations, then, that have never permeated the conscious mind and emotional impulses that have never been represented; they are merely potential psychic contents that, enduring unchanged, exert a power of "attraction" (of meaning) in relation to past experiences (Riolo 2009, p. 20). This amalgamation of sensorial experiences, descriptively and structurally, is unconscious not because it is subject to processes of repression but because psychosomatic experiences that happened before the earliest structures of psychic inscription were available are considered an expression of an "unrepressed unconscious" (Mancia 2003).

DOI: 10.4324/9781003252238-3

Irene

To give an example of this complex process in which painful experiences during the first years of life are retained intact, unelaborated, with all their traumatic potential, taking shape in subsequent phases of life in various symptomatologies, I will describe the story of Irene. Since the earliest months of life, Irene, an eight year old, had experienced relational difficulties that influenced her emotional development. At first expressed as an eating problem, during a later phase, these difficulties were transformed into a learning disturbance. Like memories tied to transgenerational elements that became current in the early mother-child relationship and were expressed as feeding difficulties, the problems were transformed over time into a symptomatology different from the original, in search of a listening process and of the possibility of once and for all being gathered up and transformed into mental experiences.

In our first meeting, the mother talked of Irene's problems at school, which pertained to reading and writing. It had been decided to consult an expert because she wondered how she could help her daughter. She and her husband tried to stay close to Irene in every way, but at times they lost patience in coping with her difficulties, feeling a sense of impotence that the mother recalled having frequently experienced in relation to her daughter.

Irene was in the second grade, having initiated first grade the previous year with great enthusiasm, but after about three months, she began to display a certain uneasiness, which manifested as an apparent fear of a particular teacher and no longer wanting to go to school. Her parents had tried to help with her attendance, gently at first and later with a certain firmness, but for four months, the child would stiffen her body, vomit, and have headaches – the typical picture of children who come to be called "phobic scholars" (D'Alberton and Ambrosi 1989). Irene had then resumed going to school, but there was a coincident drop in her academic performance, and her handwriting had become shaky and almost illegible. With first grade completed, she had begun second grade with new teachers, who noticed that the child showed a certain degree of slowness in learning.

At the time of the consultation, Irene went to school cheerfully, and she was making up for being slow in some areas. Her overall performance showed both high and low grades, with many problems in spelling and with handwriting that was almost illegible, even though at times she was capable of writing well. She read slowly but with good comprehension.

In the course of the session, I had the impression that it was difficult for Irene's mother to talk about the early years of Irene's life; she seemed able to return to the child's infancy only very slowly, and had to do so little by little, continually touching on later events at school. She told me that the girl had been in day care for a year and then attended preschool willingly, even though she tended not to show affection for the teachers and not to get involved in activities. She remembered then that, even in preschool, there had been a refusal to go to school similar to what happened at the first level of elementary school; Irene had been afraid of a preschool teacher whom she described to her mother as a fairy tale monster. At that time, too, Irene seemed to be enclosed within herself; she had crying spells and refused to participate in activities. Only over time – and with a great deal of patient understanding on the part of the teacher whom she feared – was she able to get over this.

Little by little as the session unfolded, the mother slowly began to give a descriptive glimpse of her daughter's relationship with food, which the mother remembered as "terrible." Irene had been born "normally," with a normal weight, and she was breastfed until about three months of age. At this time she began to refuse eating, which lasted for some days and was coincident with an attempt at weaning. From that period onward, the baby had been forced to eat and had had every kind of problem; her weight dropped, and what became frequent hospital visits ensued. From then on, Irene had a worsening relationship with food that had lasted through the time of the latest school crisis; continuing up to the day before; she had been force-fed or followed around with a spoon to get her to eat "without her noticing." Then, from the time when she had again begun to accept her teacher and to eat in an autonomous way, her handwriting had become tremulous, and she was brought to the consultation.

Irene's mother spoke of how much she suffered at the thought that Irene seemed to be expressing a protest against her as well, not allowing her to help with her schoolwork. "I've always had a sense of impotence with my daughter," she said,

> of not being able to nurture her, even though in reality we got on well together, and from the time she was little, Irene let me know when she needed cuddling. This year's teachers, too, describe her as a child with good prospects, but one who is isolated and anxious.

When I asked to hear more about Irene's early developmental stages, her mother recounted that, when Irene was three months old, the mother had resumed working, entrusting the baby to a babysitter in the mornings. Irene had then started to eat "in fits and starts." She had her first feeding of the day with her mother, taking in about three or four tablespoons of milk; later in the day, the babysitter struggled to feed her, and in the evening the baby refused almost everything, to the point that they had resorted to making her eat by slipping a spoon into her mouth by force. The mother concluded this part of her account by declaring, "I heard my child say 'I'm hungry' for the first time only this year."

Beginning to take into consideration the possibility that there could have been some difficulty in their relationship, the mother then returned to talking about problems with the babysitter, with whom the baby had had a good relationship; the mother began to realize that she had first unloaded Irene's difficulties onto the babysitter, then onto the school. She told about having returned to work because she wanted to get out of the house, fearing that she would otherwise not be able to detach from her daughter. She could not entrust Irene to the paternal grandparents because they lived far away, and although her own mother was nearby, Irene's mother did not have a good relationship with her and she did not want to leave the baby with her.

When I pointed out to her that she seemed to be expressing a concern about re-enacting with her daughter the same relationship that she had had with her own mother, Irene's mother agreed, and immediately afterward, she again spoke about the babysitter, whom she hadn't really liked. She had chosen her because she seemed to be experienced, but later it seemed to Irene's mother that the babysitter cuddled Irene a little too much – to the point that, after about a year, the mother thought she heard Irene call the babysitter "Mama," and she decided to find another arrangement.

The first meeting seemed characterized by a contrast between the clarity with which Irene's mother described the situation and the scant awareness of any of her own influence on the child's difficulties. In that moment, it was not possible for the mother to make any connection between her daughter's eating problems and the motives that had led her to resume teaching; or between fantasies tied to her relationship with her own mother and the motives that had led her to send away a helpful babysitter due to a fear that the child might become too attached to the babysitter; or between the symptomatic shift from anxiety about eating to academic difficulties.

At the second session, Irene's father, a young and apparently warm person, was also present. He began to speak of the recent drop in Irene's academic performance, which he did not know whether to attribute to a learning difficulty or to a lack of serious effort. As an example of his impressions, he described an episode in which the teacher had asked Irene to write a report about her fears, and she had gotten a poor grade because she had wriggled out of it by writing in two lines that she didn't have any. As was the case for Irene, also for the parents, certain feelings were at times so painful that they preferred to imagine that they didn't exist.

Trying to open up a crack in the complex system of denial that characterized the entire familial system, I alluded to the fact that sometimes it isn't easy to talk about one's fears. Almost interrupting me, the mother said that this seemed strange to her because Irene was an open child who willingly talked of what happened to her. For example, she spoke calmly about her fear of being "flunked" by her teachers.

At that moment, I found myself thinking about how similar were the parents' "being open" and Irene's "being open" – about how great was the divide between things that got said and things that were felt in relationships. While I thought about these things, Irene's mother asked me sharply – and with an attitude that I found irritating – why I was excluding the possible presence of learning problems. I answered that I did not exclude such difficulties a priori, but in that moment, it seemed to me that there were other, higher-priority factors to be thoroughly explored. I asked myself whether, behind an attitude of warmth and availability on the parents' part, there might be a veiled, intense aggression, and I reflected on how many violent acts, such as force-feeding, had been done to the little girl "for her own good." At the same time, I wondered how intensely the parents might have felt anxious and frightened about these things, and I expressed this feeling of mine to them.

Irene's mother had always felt herself annoyed with this child who didn't do things that other children did. In the course of our meeting, I tried to place myself somewhat in Irene's shoes – asking myself, together with them, what significance for her the chain of continual interruptions in close relationships that we'd talked about might have had. Could it be, perhaps, that every new close tie might represent for her the threat of a new abandonment? It didn't seem to have been by chance that, even at school, Irene's problems began after three months of attendance – just as at three months of age, she had been weaned and her mother had gone back to work. The fear of being "flunked" began to take on more meaning for the child.

When the mother told me that her daughter did not have problems saying things, that she talked a lot and was very calm, I again had a feeling that I had had many times with these parents and especially with the mother, who used a torrent of words to protect herself from a state of suffering that only very slowly began to emerge. Talking about things, describing one's own emotions, doesn't automatically mean being in contact with them.

Our conversation concluded with some reflections, which it seemed to me were shared, on the oscillation that there had been in our meeting between moments of contact and moments of distancing and on the fact that what they had felt in the session could help them understand what Irene felt when she said she was not afraid and that it could certainly be more reassuring to see her difficulty in terms of gain and of her overall comportment.

The next time, the contact that there had been seemed very far away, and the parents needed to speak to me immediately about presumed difficulties of their daughter's "lateralization." I continued to be aware that the impossibility of the parents' seeing their daughter's possible emotional disturbances irritated me and caused me to be in pain for them, feeling myself almost pushed into meeting with Irene. I found myself thinking:

> Let them bring her to see me – then we'll see if there is some specific deficit, and that way we'll all be calmer and we won't be making these parents suffer, putting them in touch with pain that they can't tolerate.

It was something of an echo of what they described to me when, in coping with their daughter's difficulties, they had felt uncertain and had oscillated between insisting that she do things, even overpowering her, and giving up in a state of resignation.

When I communicated these impressions of mine to them, Irene's mother again spoke about her own family history, and this time she recounted a series of very sad events that she had not previously mentioned. Her mother's older sister, who eventually passed away from a serious illness, had begun to get sick when Irene was three months old, and her mother's father had passed away shortly afterward.

Now the problem of three months made sense: relationships became dangerous because after a certain period of time, they were interrupted. The mother's early return to work was now equally understandable as an attempt to protect her daughter from her own mother – whom she identified with – and at the same time to protect herself from a threatened attack by death anxieties. That Irene's mother's identification with her own mother was conflictual was also apparent in her feeling that she did not have good things to give her daughter: "When it seemed to me that she had eaten enough, I said okay, that's enough, I'm hurting you, don't force yourself – and this happens now as well."

In the session, this intense exchange made me understand how much I could become, in relation to the parents, a mother who forced her children to eat bad things, painful things, and I was aware of the need to give them some breathing room. So I agreed to a series of meetings with Irene, at the end of which the parents and I would see each other again to take stock of the situation. After those meetings, we decided together to propose to Irene that she start psychotherapy with a colleague of mine, while I continued to be a referral point for the parents through periodic meetings that have continued for some years.

I think that this clinical situation lends itself to a clarification of the way that painful feelings experienced at an early age can leave behind a memory of a person's physical and mental experience – a memory that, if unheard, is dragged along over the course of generations, in a way that we will have the opportunity of exploring in depth in the chapters dedicated to parent-child consultations.

The Birth of the Mental Experience

To engage with this clinical vignette and its description of an early eating disturbance, it can be useful to refer to Eugenio Gaddini's theorizations, in particular his concepts of "fantasies in the body" and "fantasies about the body." As already mentioned, psychoanalytic thinking has historically attributed great importance to the development of fantasies through visual images that precede verbal thought. Gaddini hypothesized an earlier time in which

> primitive mental experiences of the body . . . are made up of particular sensations connected to a specific function (originally that of feeding). Where necessary, these experiences are physically expressed, actively and specifically promoting that particular function which produced those sensations which the mind has already experienced.[1]

When there are deficits in the child's environment and in the way he is cared for, the utilization of the body takes on a defensive function to guarantee the child's physical and emotional survival. These are situations that require activation of early defensive functions and where what happens at those levels remains confined within bodily experiences, without the possibility of achieving mental signification. This is something that can happen at a later time when, through the treatment and repetition of those experiences within a therapeutic relationship, the possibility can emerge of their gaining access to signification and representation, transforming the original "fantasies in the body" into "fantasies about the body."

Gaddini's thinking is rooted in a theoretical perspective that views mental experience as an evolution of the somatic-sensorial experience, of which Winnicott and Bion can be considered the precursors. This perspective can be synthesized with Winnicott's (1960) opinion that, already in the maternal womb, there is a human being in the true sense of the word – one who is capable of experiences and of accumulating bodily memories and who is even able to organize defensive measures with which to face trauma. This author describes the birth of the psyche as an imaginative elaboration of somatic components, of feelings and functions (Winnicott 1949, p. 292), emphasizing that "the True Self comes from the aliveness of the body tissues and the working of body-functions, including the heart's action and breathing."[2]

In his work "Mind and Its Relation to Psyche Soma" (1949),[3] Winnicott considers the mind to be that part of the self that takes note of what happens in experiences and connects it to the deepest part of its core. Starting from the soma, the mind forms a relationship with the body, with internal sensations, and with the external world. In other words, it makes memory (unification of past experiences) possible, as well as awareness of the current moment and expectations of the future, all connected to the individual's capacities. The mind would be born, then, out of the child's need to have a favourable environment in which he is able to develop. It would initially evolve as the part of the psyche-soma that is concerned with the relationship between the self and missing environmental elements, and it would be born from the need to give clarity to the environment at the moment in which this starts to upset the continuity of being.

The psyche-soma would evolve as part of physiological development in connection with the realization of the true self, and the mind would take care of environmental deficits in order to guarantee continuity of the individual's existence. When things go well enough, there is no great need for the mind, and the child can experience a healthy dependence on the environment. But if the environment lacks important components, or if the child is exposed to suffering that even a more appropriate environment would not be able to rescue him from, the mind is required to intervene and broaden its functions, to the detriment of harmonious development of the psyche-soma. Under these conditions, the mind tries to substitute itself for the "good enough" mother and the environment, in a way that makes them less necessary. It is a kind of self-reliance in which the mind tries to impose itself on the psyche as an "environment" and replace meaningful objects with itself.

Thus, the mind is installed as a "foreign body" in a psyche-soma that is not in contact with what happens at a deeper level, giving rise to what Winnicott defines as a seduction of the psyche on the part of the mind. The memory of failed environments, the rupture of the intimate relationship between psyche and soma that results, and the hegemony of the mind to which the individual has had to resort to protect himself from the rupture of the continuity of existence – all these continue to maintain a grip on the individual's life through the repetition of pathological conditions that have at their roots the incapacity to trust others.

Another basic contribution to our understanding of the human ability to access thinking and mental representations, to which I have alluded in the preceding chapter, is that of Wilfred Bion and other authors in the post-Bionian tradition. Among these authors in Italy, first and foremost are Antonino Ferro (2002, 2007) and Giuseppe Civitarese (2011).

Bion (1962a, 1962b) began from the basic observation that in the early phases of life, the human being, for its physical survival, needs the presence of someone who cares for him from both a physical and a mental point of view. The necessity of someone who takes care of his physical needs is directly apparent, whereas less in evidence is the early necessity of mental closeness for the development of the baby's mind, when in the primitive mind what begins to emerge from the somatic are elements that we could call *protosensations* and *protoemotions*. These are primitive emotions and primitive sensations still devoid of a mental quality, around which attempts at early thoughts are organized and which begin to associate fragments of mental images and sensations tied to somatic states into a kind of *protothinking*.

Somatic and emotional tensions linked to sensations and unsatisfied needs can represent elements that are too difficult to be processed – "indigestible" elements, that is, which the child cannot tolerate within himself and of which he tends to rid himself, principally by evacuating them, externalizing them. For example, the child rids himself of these through an experience of gratification, when anger and frustration arising from an unsatisfied need are submerged within the experience of satisfactory feeding, through which the mother absorbs, filters, and decontaminates the child's emotions. In this way, somatic and primitive emotional, "undigested" states can be transformed so that, in place of indigestible and intractable feelings, an area of acceptance and satisfaction is created. A theory of thinking follows from this, one in which the experience connected to sensorial, protoemotional states (beta elements) can be thinkable, at either a conscious or unconscious level, only if it is transformed into basic representations (alpha elements) through the work of a psychic function designated the *alpha function*.

With reverie, the mother places her own alpha function into the service of the child's still immature one. Thanks to this maternal function, the child is helped to decontaminate his internal reality, to transform it into conceivable and representable elements. In time, he finds a way to make this capacity his own and to carry out this function independently.

Both Winnicott and Bion are considered pillars of a kind of bridge between English psychoanalysis – or object relations – and French psychoanalysis – more focused on the concept of the drive. A particularly creative attempt to hold these two theoretical approaches together is found in a work by René Roussillon (1999), which dedicates careful consideration to the metapsychological mandate of processes of symbolization, a term he uses to try to explain the birth of mental life and the development of thinking. He describes the evolution of subjective experience, what is, the modalities in which primary sensorial experiences are registered in psychic life through their inscription in "psychic vestiges." His starting point is represented by what Freud called early "psychic material" and the modalities with which it is assigned to mental experiences (Freud 1900, p. 496). Roussillon (2017) is describing, in other words, the complexity of sensations that various sources of sensoriality and perception propagate in the psyche through motility, at a substantially unconscious level.

Symbolization – and more in general representational activity – would take its origins from the absence of the object, and it would have to do with the way in which an absent object can continue to maintain its psychic presence through psychic vestiges of previous perceptions. In the early phases of life, it is believed that a type of primary symbolization takes place that depends in large part on the baby's early relationships with the surrounding environment, which has been described in various ways. For example, Piera Aulagnier (1975) and Antonino Ferro (2002), in different ways, have spoken of pictograms; Didier Anzieu (1975) of formal meanings; Jean Laplanche (1987) of enigmatic meanings – all attempts to describe the initial primitive experiences of subjective appropriation of reality, anchored in the body's sensorimotor aspects and its sensoriality.

For Roussillon, following Freud, symbolic representation incorporates a vestige of the work of a reflexive movement that presents it and recognizes it as a *psychic representation* and sets things up so that it is subjectively presented as a representation, not a perception. The work that undergoes early registration in order to be considered a "representation" and then a "symbolic representation" comes to be designated the *work of symbolization*, through which the representation is conceived as a new internal presentation that allows processes of thinking to occur and can reach consciousness. Just as Freud proposed two modalities of thinking – *primary process* of unconscious experiences themselves and *secondary process*, typical of more developed experiences of thinking – Roussillon proposes *primary symbolization* and *secondary symbolization*. The first, connected to transformation at the unconscious level of a "mnestic perceptive trace," would be represented substantially at an unconscious level, as though it were a thing (thing representation), and the second, adding early forms of linguistic connotation, would lead to the ability to utilize it psychically as a "word representation," approaching thought processes with preconscious and conscious characteristics. Roussillon expresses some doubt about the existence of presymbolic memories; in order to be remembered, a memory would have to have some form of representation, even though primary or at a level of "representation of a perception" (Golse and Roussillon 2010, p. 26).

What I have related describes attempts to provide some hypotheses about the birth of the psychic world, about the passage from perception to memory and thinking, during periods in which it is difficult to speak of thinking and memory in organisms that are still equipped with basic neuronal structures.

An example that well describes the passage from a level of primary symbolization to one of secondary symbolization can be seen in the person who, over many years, has not been able to explain why certain sounds – such as, for example, a microwave oven beep – cause him to feel uneasy. Only with the distance of many years – and to his great surprise – was this man capable of connecting the beep that caused him discomfort to crib alarms that he happened to hear on a recent visit to the neonatal hospital unit where he himself had spent long periods of time as an infant.

Psychoanalysis and Neuroscience

It appears that the field of neuroscience can shed new light on the early phases of existence – in that, although it draws on its own epistemological references and realms, as does psychoanalysis, neuroscience observes from different perspectives the same object: the human being (Spagnolo 2018). Readings from this discipline should not be ruled out as irrelevant, but on the contrary, they can offer reciprocal confirmations, as Schore maintains: "Neuropsychoanalytic studies of the evolution of psychic structure attempt to more deeply understand the essential psychological processes and biological mechanisms that underlie the psychobiological substrate of the human unconscious described by Freud."[4]

For example, it is interesting to note that scientific experiments have led Siegel to affirm how much psychoanalysis has long been supported at an empirical level. New-born infants perceive the environment that surrounds them from the earliest days of life, and various studies have demonstrated that even very young infants are capable of having earlier memories, which are manifested in terms of behavioural, perceptive, and emotional learning (Siegel 1999, p. 28).

From other research, we learn that, in the short term, the memory of painful experiences influences behaviours in very young children and permanently lowers the threshold of pain and the activation of psycho-endocrinological mechanisms in response to stress. This is thanks to areas of research that view psychosomatic experience as able to influence both the stability of synaptic connections between neurons and the programming of neurochemical responses that can impact the total organism (Balbernie 2001).

In fact, Schore maintains that the parents' competence in being tuned in to the child's mental state and his early experiences of attachment play an essential role in the development and maturation of cerebral circuits that determine the capacity for self-regulation. Schore believes that the orbitofrontal system of the right brain constitutes the hierarchical apex of the limbic system and the autonomous system; in other words, it is the most active cerebral apparatus capable of regulating stress that arises within the relational context characterizing early relationships. During a critical period for the maturation of the orbitofrontal cortex, elevated levels of stress hormones can compromise the early organization and connections of the prefrontal system, charged with non-conscious processing of the information that connects external, objectual relational indices with internal bodily states (Schore

2003, p. 376). Neuroscience, then, confirms that: "Cerebral circuits 'remember' and learn from past experiences through a growing probability of reaching determined patterns of activation" (Siegel 1999, p. 24, translation by G. Atkinson).

There are two types of memory implicated in these processes: *procedural memory* and autobiographical, *declarative memory*. Procedural memory, with its early component – implicit, not declarative – is juxtaposed to and integrated with an explicit, declarative memory to be developed later, involving evocative autobiographical and semantic competencies (Squire 1994; Schacter and Tulving 1994). Conscious awareness of our personal history is based on explicit memory; here memories are tied to words, are more or less directly retrievable, and mental images are imagined and can be recalled under certain conditions. Associated with the common experience of a conscious recollection, it is this type of memory to which we turn in order to recognize the continuity of our experience in time, to locate episodes and instances of learning in our lives that require focused attention. Its utilization requires the maturation of cerebral structures to be developed at a later point, such as the medial temporal lobe, the region of the hippocampus, and the orbitofrontal cortex.

Implicit procedural memory, on the other hand, refers to experiences that pertain to emotions present before the child is capable of utilizing a psychic apparatus that allows him to "think thoughts" (Bion 1962b), to give names to the sensations that he experiences. This involves the possibility of transcribing experiences that have taken place prior to development of the capacity to make use of symbols or language, which requires the maturation of more developed brain structures. The cerebral structures and circuits of procedural memory, it is believed, involve the posterior temporo-parieto-occipital areas of the right hemisphere and amygdala. These memories influence our way of predicting, anticipating, and living relationships, of which one has a lived experience but without the possibility of directly recalling them to conscious mentation. It is this type of memory, it is hypothesized, that allows the new-born infant to hold early experiences inside himself.

This dimension of implicit memory can relate to the final periods of gestational life as well, in which the foetus lives in very close relationship with the mother – with her rhythms (cardiac and respiratory) and her voice (Mancia 1981, p. 351). Recent studies suggest that even if early painful memories are not accessible to conscious evocation, they can be codified in the "procedural memory" that leads to altered models of behaviour or sensorial activities in subsequent life (Anand and Scalzo 2000, p. 71).

In regard to the memory of processes of symbolization, Stefano Calamandrei recalls Modell's attempt to find connections between psychoanalytic theories and neuroscientific findings, formulating the hypothesis that the unrepressed unconscious may be the area in which utilization of the metaphor can take place. Metaphorical thought would assume the basic function of interpreting the unconscious memory of somatic sensations precisely because emotional memories form categories based on metaphorical similitude. The unrepressed unconscious, then, is composed of symbols that have been unconventionally shaped by the bodily imagination, which generates innumerable proto-metaphors that have a tendency, in turn, to converge and structure themselves into primary metaphors that mould basic cognitive tools (Calamandrei 2017, p. 194).

To give another example of this passage from the biological to the mental as it pertains to memory, I will present some excerpts from the clinical story of a child who, at two and one-half years, was not able to feed himself solid food.

Luigi

A consultation about Luigi had been requested because of a "suspected psychological delay in a child born prematurely, with investigations in progress for esophageal gastric reflux." According to the father, the child's suffering was due to the use of a nasogastric probe with which he had been fed while in an incubator as an infant. In the father's opinion, this had caused a lesion that continued to cause pain even now. In fact, when Luigi was born at around the thirtieth week, he weighed less than two and a half pounds and spent more than a month being tube-fed in an incubator.

Now almost three years old, Luigi walked, talked, had acquired bowel control, and had been attending preschool for a while. But although he could bite, he was unable to feed himself solid food, and even a small lump of cheese caused him to retch. He seemed interested in food while his parents were eating, at times picking up his spoon and taking it to his mouth, but then he would stop, as though caution prevailed over curiosity. His recent introduction to preschool seemed to have gone well for three weeks, up until his current hospitalization.

While the mother asked herself how, as parents, they could have gone wrong to cause their son to establish such a negative relationship with food, the father remembered the baby's expression as he tried to swallow with the feeding tube, and the mere memory of those moments brought back to the father a pain that he reexperienced somatically as well; it made his flesh creep. According to him, Luigi seemed in his first three months of life to be wracked by painful sensations in the digestive tract – before, during, and after being fed – which almost never allowed him to sleep at night.

At first, I let myself be convinced by this hypothesis, and I imagined that the pain due to reflux and esophagitis justified the symptomatology. I understood the physical pain to be so intense that, when the father reported that Luigi even avoided touching his mouth (which he had never used in exploratory play), a passage from the gospel of Matthew went through my mind:

> If your hand or your foot causes you to stumble, cut it off and throw it away. It is better for you to enter life maimed or crippled than to have two hands or two feet and be thrown into eternal fire.
>
> (Matthew 18:8)

Luigi's parents appeared to be very attached to him and thus united with him in his suffering, and for fear of making him suffer even more, they seemed incapable of setting limits on his behaviour, even when it was necessary. Descriptions of other episodes that gradually came to light caused me to wonder if, behind the real suffering that the child felt, a distortion of the relationship might have been allowing him to manipulate his parents according to his own desires. Especially the attitude of the father – who on the ward was called "Mr. Mom" – and who appeared affectionate, concerned, and close to his son, made me think that one of the problems might be excessive attempts to try to satisfy the little boy's needs.

In spite of our fantasies, the eventual results of examinations of oesophageal acidity and the digestive tube excluded both reflux and esophagitis, and the therapy aimed at attenuating such pains was suspended. "There's something I don't understand," the father said at one point. "Why did Luigi stop eating cereal, when before he used to eat it? He should be eating it again now, if the pain we thought was there actually isn't."

I thought about saying that maybe the pain was there, even if it wasn't only physical, and that contact with something hard, something different from the consistency of foods he was familiar with, could have caused him to have strange sensations that scared him. I had the impression that for Luigi, the role of a border between internal and external, normally played by the skin, had in some way shifted to the digestive tract – as though, in place of instinctual feelings of hunger and satisfaction, the oesophagus had become a sensitive zone around which an early, rudimentary differentiation was organized between the internal and the external of the body.

As we will see more clearly in a later chapter devoted to parent-child consultations, the experience of becoming a parent ushers into the familial scene the parents' personal history and experiences, as well as their childhood relationships with their own parents. Sometimes these family stories bring with them a fear of reactivating episodes of suffering that occurred when they themselves were children – often events tied to aggression and distance in relationships – and the desire not to re-enact this with the child can be quite strong.

It would seem that Luigi's parents might have been unprepared for the birth of a real child – so different from the child of their imagination, who would be "handled with kid gloves" and would need only to be kept content. The neonatal experience had been especially traumatic for them; it had crystallized around the memory of the "probe," which had probably impaired their ability to bear the difficulties tied to all the forms of weaning and had not allowed them to move from an insurmountable physical pain to a manageable psychic pain. This was a story in which the parents, traumatized by the experience of neonatal problems, may have too closely identified with their son, and they had not been able to represent to him with sufficient confidence the fact that even very painful transitory experiences could be assimilated, digested.

Painful bodily sensations felt during a period in which they could not be transformed into thinkable forms and a way of processing them that divided them into good or bad could subsequently have given rise to a stark contrast between soft foods and solid foods, in which the quality of solid food came to represent what had been strange and could not be assimilated.

Marco La Scala (2017) helps us understand these situations when he revisits the concept of pictograms proposed by Piera Aulagnier, which we've already touched on briefly. La Scala characterizes this term as one that lends itself to describing the meeting between a sensorial zone and its complementary object. The mouth meets the breast and between them a mirror-like refraction occurs, which becomes the prototype of a meeting based on complementarity and reciprocal co-penetration (La Scala 2017, p. 84). La Scala quotes from Aulagnier[5]:

> Every organ of pleasure, however, can become precisely what one mutilates oneself with in order to cancel out the displeasure for which one is suddenly shown to be responsible. . . . The "rejection" outside the self is first illustrated by the creation of a reciprocal rejection between zone and object. . . . The desire to destroy the object will always be accompanied in its original form by the desire to annihilate an erotic and sensorial zone, as well as the activity of which this zone is the central location.
>
> (Aulagnier 1975, pp. 92–93, translation by G. Atkinson)

For Luigi, the internal hell, the very painful experience that made it difficult for him to nurture himself, was the originary experience of the meeting with the object that exposed him to an anxiety harkening back to a condition of impotence. The prototype of this impotence consists of the psychosomatic states tied to the sudden passage from intrauterine life to life outside the womb. This is a sharp interruption in the homeostasis of foetal conditions, in which "the stable and constant limit of the amniotic membrane, reinforced by the uterine wall, is now missing" (Gaddini 1981, p. 481, translation by G. Atkinson). Through the treatment systems that surround the baby, giving him the impression that something or someone is taking care of him and protecting him from reliving those primitive sensations of impotence and disorganization of internal and external stimuli, there is a gradual reconstruction of the earlier homeostatic condition.

The importance of positive experiences within early relationships is reinforced by Schore (2003), who, locating himself in the realm of psychoanalytic thinking, in line with theoreticians of different psychoanalytic traditions – Bion, Winnicott, and Kohut – states that: "In critical early periods of life, the brain-mind-body system of the growing human being is developed through systems of ever greater complexity in the context of a relationship, for affective regulation, with another human being" (p. 28, translation by G. Atkinson).

Repetition, day after day and hour after hour, of the experience of being cared for, in which tense situations give way to a lack of tension and to satisfaction, sets up the conditions in which the experience of trust can be solidified. We can imagine, then, that the greater the good experiences, the greater the possibility that the quality of the experience will be characterized by positive feelings, by a sense of basic trust (Erikson 1950), by a sense of well-being and security (Sandler 1960). Prolonged painful experiences, a lack of care, or unsatisfied instinctual needs seem to lead in the opposite direction.

Freud hypothesized that the psychic apparatus mobilizes defences against the perception that provokes anxiety (1925) and that painful stimuli are treated by the psychic apparatus as foreign elements obstructing the process of symbolization that we talked about earlier. Other authors highlight the existence of proto-defensive behaviours formed during a preverbal period, which do not express internal conflicts but rather the attempt to avoid awareness of painful affects (Bastianini and Moccia 2003, p. 533).

We can imagine that Luigi's parents did not have sufficient tools to help him come out of those painful states – that past suffering in their own personal histories continued to influence the parental experience. Only a process of psychic working through of those primitive painful experiences can permit Luigi to accept the limits of his desires; and, as we will see in subsequent chapters, this will help his future offspring cope with physical and mental pain connected to growing up for what it actually is. Thus the intergenerational continuation of an un-worked-through memory of these experiences will be avoided, through the specified ways of protecting against their continuing to be dragged along in the chain of generations.

Conclusions

This chapter began with the question of whether it is possible for the child to forget memories of early painful experiences or avoid having these influence him in his subsequent life. We have seen how difficult that is, even if the overall developmental journey offers opportunities to integrate suffering and limit its influence. To summarize what has been previously stated, the development of the self in the new-born infant unfolds through bodily sensations. Such development coalesces around positive sensations connected to the satisfaction of emotional and instinctual needs, which early on are split apart from negative or painful sensations tied to neediness, to frustration, to pain. All that is good shapes the self, in contrast to the non-self, which begins to be characterized as composed of negative experiences.

On the one hand, processes of negation and of splitting off negative experiences fulfil a protective function with respect to painful experiences that go beyond the mind's capacity to contain them. On the other hand, when an excess of these defences is set in motion, they risk limiting the encounter with the global range of feelings and the complexity of existence. In addition, because the quality of these early experiences influences the development of the encephalitic structures themselves, prenatal development and the first two years of life are the period in which genetic foundations are created – organic and neurochemical – for the control of impulses and emotions.

But if all that is true, we might spontaneously ask ourselves why the belief may have taken hold that the small child, due to the immaturity of his organs and primordial systems of communication, does not retain a memory of pain. I think that at play here are protective factors with respect to the intensity of anxiety that one feels when encountering a child who is suffering. In the meeting with the infant – who is such precisely because he is an *infant*, that is, he doesn't speak – the non-verbal expression of pain evokes in the adult who comes into contact – and also in ourselves as clinical caregivers, an echo of ancient suffering – pain without a name and without words that can resonate with similar experiences to which we may have been exposed in our own childhoods. We are called upon to find a reasonable balance between those who deny the baby's pain and those who – like Luigi's parents – take it into maximal consideration without being able to imagine that a traumatic and painful experience, with adequate support, can be transformed into an experience of growth.

"It's something bad that gets forgotten," "crying makes the eyes beautiful," "crying strengthens the lungs," "the baby won't remember the pain" – these are cultural platitudes that our society employs almost to exorcise the difficulty of being in contact with children's pain and anxiety. As professionals, we cannot ask ourselves to live the pain being expressed in that moment with the same intensity as the parent or the child whom we are treating. Perhaps, however, we can acknowledge to ourselves that the pain, though evoking deep and anguished emotions, can be taken into account, not denied, without that implying the breakdown of the adaptive defence system that is necessary in personal and professional terms in order to be in contact with situations of such great emotional intensity, such as those at the border between life and non-life, connected to painful episodes experienced in the early phases of life.

Notes

1   Gaddini, E. (1981). Early defensive fantasies and the psychoanalytical process. In *A Psychoanalytic Theory of Infantile Experience: Conceptual and Clinical Reflections*, ed. A. Limentani. London: Institute of Psychoanalysis, 1992, p. 125.
2   Winnicott, D. W. (1960). Ego distortion in terms of true and false self. In *The Maturational Processes and the Facilitating Environment: Studies in the Theory of Emotional Development*. London: The Hogarth Press and the Institute of Psychoanalysis, 1965, p. 148.
3   In *Collected Papers*. London: Tavistock, 1958.
4   Schore, A. N. (2011). The right brain implicit self lies at the core of psychoanalysis. *Psychoanal. Dialogues*, 21:75–100, p. 75.
5   Aulagnier, P. (1975). *The Violence of Interpretation: From Pictogram to Statement*, trans. A. Sheridan. London: Institute of Psychoanalysis, 2001, pp. 92–93.

References

Anand, K. J. S. & Scalzo, F. M. (2000). Can adverse neonatal experiences alter brain development and subsequent behavior? *Neonatology*, 77:69–82.

Anzieu, D. (1975). La psychanalyse encore. *Revue Français de Psychanalyse.*, 1(2):135–146.

Aulagnier, P. (1975). *The Violence of Interpretation: From Pictogram to Statement*, trans. A. Sheridan. London: Institute of Psychoanalysis, 2001.

Balbernie, R. (2001). Circuits and circumstances: The neurobiological consequences of early relationship experiences and how they shape later behaviour. *J. Child Psychother.*, 27:237–255.

Bastianini, T. & Moccia, G. (2003). Riflessioni sulle attuali evoluzioni dei concetti di affetto, memoria e azione terapeutica [Reflections on current developments in the concepts of affect, memory, and therapeutic action]. *Rivista di Psicoanalisi*, 49:529–549.

Bion, W. R. (1962a). A theory of thinking. In *Second Thoughts*. New York: Jason Aronson, 1967, pp. 110–119.

———. (1962b). *Learning from Experience*. London: Routledge, 1984.

Calamandrei, S. (2017). *L'Identità creativa: Psicoanalisi e neuroscienze del pensiero simbolico e metaforico [Creative Identity: Psychoanalysis and Neurosciences of Symbolic and Metaphorical Thinking]*. Milano: FrancoAngeli.

Civitarese, G. (2011). *The Violence of Emotions: Bion and Post-Bionian Psychoanalysis*. London: New Library of Psychoanalysis, 2012.

D'Alberton, F. & Ambrosi, S. (1989). Riflessi sul rifiuto della scuola a partire dal concetto nosografico di "fobia scolare" [Reflections on the refusal of school starting from the nosographical concept of "school girl phobia"]. *Psichiatria dell'infanzia e dell'adolescenza*, 56:427–446.

Erikson, E. H. (1950). *Childhood and Society*. New York: Norton.

Ferro, A. (2002). *Seeds of Illness, Seeds of Recovery*, trans. P. Slotkin. Hove, UK: Brunner-Routledge, 2005.

———. (2007). *Avoiding Emotions, Living Emotions*, trans. I. Harvey. London: New Library of Psychoanalysis, 2011.

Freud, S. (1900). The interpretation of dreams. *S. E.*, 4/5.

———. (1925). Inhibitions, symptoms, and anxiety. *S. E.*, 20.

Gaddini, E. (1981). Early defensive fantasies and the psychoanalytical process. In *A Psychoanalytic Theory of Infantile Experience: Conceptual and Clinical Reflections*, ed. A. Limentani. London: Institute of Psychoanalysis, 1992.

Golse, B. & Roussillon, R. (2010). *La Naissance de l'objet*. Paris: Presses Universitaires Française.

Laplanche, J. (1987). *New Foundations for Psychoanalysis*, trans. D. Macey. Cambridge, MA/Oxford, UK: Basil Blackwell, 1989.

La Scala, M. (2017). *Percepire, allucinare, immaginare [Perceiving Hallucinating, Imagining]*. Milano: FrancoAngeli.

Mancia, M. (1981). On the beginning of mental life in the foetus. *Int. J. Psychoanal.*, 62:351–357.

———. (2003). Implicit memory and unrepresssed unconscious: Their role in creativity and transference. *Israel Psychoanal. J.*, 3:331–349.

Riolo, F. (2009). Lo statuto psicoanalitico di inconscio. *Rivista di Psicoanalisi*, 55, 1:11–28.

Roussillon, R. (1999). *Agonie, clivage et symbolisation*. Paris: Presses Universitaires Française.

———. (2017). Fondamenti e processi dell'incontro psicoanalitico [Foundations and Processes of the Psychoanalytic Encounter]. In *La relazione psicoanalitica: Contributi clinici e teorici [The Psychoanalytic Relationship: Clinical and Theoretical Contributions]*, ed. N. Rossi & I. Ruggiero. Milano: FrancoAngeli.

Sandler, J. (1960). The background of safety. *Int. J. Psychoanal.*, 41:352–356.

Schacter, D. L. & Tulving, E., eds. (1994). *Memory Systems*. Cambridge, MA: MIT Press.

Schore, A. N. (2003). *Affect Regulation and Repair of the Self*. New York: Norton.

———. (2011). The right brain implicit self lies at the core of psychoanalysis. *Psychoanal. Dialogues*, 21:75–100.

Siegel, D. J. (1999). *The Developing Mind: Toward a Neurobiology of Interpersonal Experience*. New York: Guilford Press.

Spagnolo, R., ed. (2018). *Building Bridges: The Impact of Neuropsychoanalysis on Psychoanalytic Clinical Sessions*. London: Routledge.

Squire, L. R. (1994). Declarative and non-declarative memory: Multiple brain systems supporting learning and memory. In *Memory Systems*, ed. D. L. Schacter & E. Tulving. Cambridge, MA: MIT Press, pp. 203–232.

Winnicott, D. W. (1949). Mind and its relation to psyche soma. In *Collected Papers*. London: Tavistock, 1958.

———. (1960). The theory of the parent-infant relationship. In *The Maturational Processes and the Facilitating Environment: Studies in the Theory of Emotional Development*. London: Routledge, 1984.

Chapter 3

The Different Times of Trauma and Its Intergenerational Transmission

Seated across from me, the parents of four-year-old Ivan are trying to find the best way to bring the child up to date about the physical problem that has brought him to the hospital and the surgical intervention that he will soon undergo. While we talk, Ivan is in his father's arms, immersed in what seems to be a deep sleep. After I have listened at length, I speak to them, turning to Ivan as well, taking it for granted that he is listening to me and knowing how useful it can be for children to be involved, informed, and able to think about what pertains to them.

Some time after the beginning of our meeting, Ivan opens one eye and then the other, and, giving the impression of one who has decided that he can trust me and trust this place, he slides off his dad's lap and begins to explore the environment that surrounds him, heading toward a box of games in a little space behind me reserved for children. Ivan's mother appears somewhat surprised; she asks me if it's okay to make games available to children because, in her opinion, games can serve a protective function but can also interfere with understanding things. This statement is a little strange in reference to a four-year-old child and, more than trying to follow its logic, I look for the reasons behind the mother's concern.

My curiosity is aroused by the mother's observation, to which it would be just as simple as it was useless to give a reply such as: it isn't necessary to have studied advanced psychology to know that children think while they are playing; they play spontaneously and, through their play, they spontaneously express emotions and fantasies about the characters who inhabit their internal world. Psychoanalysis, on the other hand, has helped us understand that if a person expresses a thought that clashes with the usual way of thinking, it is most often not because of ignorance or cultural or intellectual limitations but because a glimmer of unconscious emotional contents is opening up – contents that tend to head off toward some form of mental representation, even if bizarre.

I decide to probe that small opening, and I ask the mother what leads her to think that playing could have the effect on her son that she fears. From that moment on, it is as though another session begins. She moves her chair and positions herself between me and the child, with a change of perspective that places her in the foreground; she does not seem to be a parent talking about her son, but rather it

DOI: 10.4324/9781003252238-4

is as though a child part of the mother has entered the scene and asks to be heard. She tells about having suffered sexual abuse at the age of four, which she became aware of only at age nineteen, noting as well that during that entire period, she had continued to utilize games and fantasies almost as a way to seal up her mind and keep herself from realizing what had happened.

The memory of what had occurred and that took shape as a traumatic experience had continued to exist and to carry out its action inside her, without the mother herself being aware of it – if only in the form of a vague disquiet when, concomitant with her first romantic experiences, boys began to approach her, and she didn't understand why she had the feeling that they were taking advantage of her, "even if they loved me."

Some years later, following an affective experience with someone older than she who held a managerial role in the company she worked for and who had demonstrated an interest in her, an episode from her childhood came to her mind in which a family friend had approached her, brought her to a secluded place, restrained her, and touched her genitals. She had started to cry without really understanding what was happening and without being able to tell her parents what she had experienced.

At age nineteen, once the memory of that episode was made available to her conscious mind, many things had assumed significance for her. She had spoken of them to her mother, who remembered perfectly well the afternoon when she had come home crying. The mother had accepted in good faith the explanation provided by the family friend, who said that the child had suddenly become frightened, whereas the child herself was not in a position to give her own version of what had happened.

This clinical account of what took place at our first and only meeting seems a good starting point for a consideration of the different facets of trauma and its various temporalities, in order to highlight how, even in hospital work, it may be possible to experience the validity of the conceptual psychoanalytic set-up and its particular listening attitude that lends itself to multiple uses, even outside the analytic office.

Time, Trauma, Relationship

Theorizing trauma kept Freud busy for the entire course of his life and continues to pique our interest even today, eluding our attempts to reduce the concept to unequivocal definitions. Freudian thinking about trauma seems to be mapped out along two general theoretical lines, the first primarily quantitative and economic and the second qualitative and structural. In my opinion, Freud shows a decisive preference for the economic aspect, as evident in one of his more detailed definitions:

> Indeed, the term "traumatic" has no other sense than an economic one. We apply it to an experience which within a short period of time presents the mind with an increase of stimulus too powerful to be dealt with or worked

off in the normal way, and this must result in permanent disturbances of the manner in which the energy operates.

[Freud 1917, p. 275]

But this same definition contains within it an almost irreconcilable contradiction between quantitative aspects and qualitative/relational ones, which is not successfully overcome even by subsequent definitions – such as that of Laplanche and Pontalis (1973), which describes trauma as:

An event in the subject's life defined by its intensity, by the subject's incapacity to respond adequately to it, and by the upheaval and long-lasting effects that it brings about in the psychical organisation.

In economic terms, the trauma is characterised by an influx of excitations that is excessive by the standard of the subject's tolerance and capacity to master such excitations and work them out psychically.

[p. 465]

On the one hand it is precisely the intensity of stimuli – and on the other the capabilities of the psychic apparatus to process them – that determines their placement in a "complementary series" of factors between individual constitution and life experiences (Freud 1915).

Freud thought that the psychic apparatus could cope with only a certain amount of energy and that a trauma begins to take shape when an influx of excitations goes beyond the subject's ability to psychically elaborate them – that is, to connect them to mental representations. Over time, *the function of the protective shield* (1925) assumed importance in his thinking, that is, the parents' function in protecting the child from an excess of simulation. Freud did not renounce either of his two theories, and the two models coexist in his thinking almost as though to underline the dual nature of the traumatic experience, the quantitative and the relational, which can assume major or minor importance according to the observational vertex.

I think one cannot but agree with Baranger et al. (1988) when they observe that:

The distinction between external traumatic situations due to the effective absence of the object, the increment of external stimuli, etc., and of the internal stimuli due to the increase in the tensions of needs or in the drive tensions, tends to disappear since, whatever the origin of the traumatic situation, it leads to an "overwhelming" of the ego, which is unable to handle this traumatic situation that reactivates its primitive state of "helplessness."

[1988, p. 118]

Dimensions of Trauma

The various implicit aspects of the concept of trauma have led Bokanowski (2005) to distinguish three different meanings. He utilizes the term *traumatism* to define "a level of disorganisation that has more to do with secondary processes – one that does not disrupt object relations or the binding of the instinctual drives" (p. 252). He refers to the sexual traumatism of the theory of infantile sexuality that, in his early period of theorizing, Freud thought was always present when trauma occurs.

Bokanowski designates the term *trauma* to describe "a phenomenon which operates at a more primitive and less developed stage; here, the harmful effects may jeopardise narcissistic cathexes and therefore the organisation of the ego itself" (ibid). Finally, he makes use of the term *traumatic* to define "a pattern of mental functioning which is common to both of these variants and which is related to that aspect of the traumatic impact that involves the compulsion to repeat" (ibid). Furthermore, according to this author, from a chronological point of view, the conceptualization of trauma seems to take shape during three time periods in the development of Freud's thinking. He lays out these periods as between 1895 and 1897, around 1920, and 1938 – periods in which theoretical changes emerge concerning the nature, quality, and objective of traumatism in relation to psychic functioning.

During the first period, from 1895 to 1920, as indicated earlier, trauma came to be thought of as a consequence of infantile seduction, which – in a dual-time dynamic – led to the memory of events becoming pathogenic. When these events took place, they did not have a traumatic effect. Through "neurotic" revision (Freud 1887–1904), the influence of the reality of infantile seduction came to be re-dimensioned and, in the light of his discoveries about infantile sexuality, Freud brought to the foreground the role of fantasy and unconscious phantasms.

In a later period, starting in 1920, traumatism was connected to the lack of a para-excitatory shield – that is, an overall level of parental care that avoids bringing the child into contact with a quantity of stimuli that are excessive for him (Freud 1925). Traumatic neurosis, through the compulsion to repeat, is the expression of the child's impotence in the face of a quantitatively excessive stimulation in relation to the capacity of his psychic apparatus to cope with it.

In the third period, at the end of his work – in *Moses and Monotheism* (1939) – Freud (1934–1939) unifies the conception of traumatism, connecting it to narcissism; the point at which a narcissistic wound causes a trauma can influence psychic functioning and its organization.

Trauma and *Nachträglichkeit*

The concept of *Nachträglichkeit*, translated in English by *deferred action* and by the more felicitous *après-coup* in French – another important polysemic Freudian intuition (1895, 1896, 1918), one that is closely interwoven with that of trauma – opened new avenues for understanding its temporal dimensions. According to Birksted-Breen (2003), this concept, historically presented almost as a division between Anglophone psychoanalysis and Francophone psychoanalysis, was utilized by Freud with various meanings that she summarizes with the following:

The first simply means "subsequent."

The second implies movement that goes from the past to the future: in the individual, something is deposited that will be activated only later on, according to the model of the seduction theory in which the trauma is formed in two phases.

The third meaning implies the idea that the experience may have found a representation, a psychic inscription that assumes meaning only retrospectively in psychic experiences that can then give way to a form of awareness.

Like trauma, *Nachträglichkeit*, too, has followed Freud's cultural journey from start to finish; and for this concept as well, rethinking and re-elaboration have continued to operate alongside the initial formulations. A line of continuity in Freud's thinking – stretching from his letters to Fliess (Freud 1887–1902) and *Project for a Scientific Psychology* (1895) to works that conclude the trajectory of his opus, *Constructions in Analysis* (1937b), *Analysis Terminable and Interminable* (1937a), and *Moses and Monotheism* (1939) – can be seen in the many subsequent works on *Nachträglichkeit*.[1]

According to Ferraro and Garella (2009), the evolution of the concept of *Nachträglichkeit* also follows a temporal cadence at three points in the flow of Freud's thinking – "with three high points" or "three intense moments of theoretical elaboration." An innovative concentration of lines of thought is almost superimposed onto the three noteworthy temporal periods of elaboration of the concept of trauma identified by Bokanowski: that between 1895 and 1897, around 1920, and around 1938.

In the first period, starting from 1895, the traumatic action of seduction in determining neuroses – connected at first to the real experience of seduction and subsequently to infantile sexual fantasies and to unconscious phantasms – takes on traumatic meaning when physical development and mental development permit the meaning of what happened to be grasped.

In the second period, 1914–1918, around the time of the draft and publication of "The Wolf Man" (1918), posteriority is seen as "a formative trait of psychic reality, normal and pathological" (Ferraro and Garella 2009, p. 106, translation by G. Atkinson).

Between 1934 and 1938, in the third period, in *Moses and Monotheism*, Freud at the end of his life – though not referring directly to the concept of *Nachträglichkeit* – emphasizes later periods in the determination of neurotic symptomatology, in analogy with the development of historical phenomena.

More recent discussions (Dahl 2010; Turo 2013) underline the bidirectional movement of *Nachträglichkeit* – toward the future and the past – and a more complete vision of it that includes "the repetition of deferred action of memory in the transference and its retroactive revision of meaning is at the core of the psychoanalytic process" (Turo 2013).

Nachträglichkeit and trauma therefore appear to be closely connected concepts, almost two faces of the same coin, both carriers of an intimate and irrefutable contradiction between an economic hypothesis – quantitatively connected to the intensity of the traumatic stimulus – and a structural hypothesis linked to the ability of the psychic apparatus to withstand that event.

It seems that all three of the meanings of *Nachträglichkeit* listed by Birksted-Breen and of trauma by Bokanowski are implied in the experience of Ivan's mother. First of all, this was something later on that happened at a second time with respect to a quantitatively excessive originary action, "a seductive sexual action exerted by an external object," manifested as a defect of the "parastimulus" function – that is, the lack of a protective element, which exposes the subject to anxiety at a second time of trauma as "a bomb with a delayed explosion." A lack of attention on the part of those whose task is to provide the child with emotional resonance means that only with the distance of many years does a new possibility for psychic inscription permit the repair of psychic functioning whose organization has been injured by early insults to the ego that compromise its integrity and entail wounds of a narcissistic type (Freud 1934–1938).

Trauma and Intergenerational Transmission: The New Temporality of *Nachträglichkeit*

At the time it happened, Ivan's mother seems not to have been able to assimilate and mentally represent the traumatic episode into some form of memory – and, though continuing to carry out its action and influencing her feelings in situations that could reevoke it, this form could not be transformed into a conscious thought. Her not having found an interlocutor to help her give meaning to her feelings – and her reaction of instead contenting herself with a convenient explanation – meant that the experience was relegated to a split zone of the mind and that the activities of fantasy and play had the aim of covering it up with mental images in the service of self-protection. Only at a second moment did what Freud describe take place; he stated that "affective states are incorporated into the life of the psyche as precipitates of primal traumatic experiences, and are evoked in similar situations like memory symbols" (1935, p. 622).

So it was that in adulthood, in a situation similar to the original traumatic one, it had been possible for Ivan's mother to reappropriate these feelings, giving them meaning and recognizing and expressing the emotions and affects that at that time she had not been able to take in. An analytic treatment would probably have allowed her to see the episode that happened when she was four years old as a new edition in *après-coup* of an excess of earlier sensorial stimulations or of a lack of emotional attunement on the part of her parents (Freud 1918; Laplanche 1987).

And the traumatic operation that was now part of this woman's experience did not end with the original personal event; once she in turn became a mother, in a kind of identification with the aggressor (A. Freud 1936), in line with a new dimension of *Nachträglichkeit*, she wasn't able to support her son's experience in coping with a difficult moment of his development – namely, the surgical intervention from which Ivan had defensively taken refuge in sleep in order to avoid thinking about something that seemed to him impossible to talk about.

For a parent, the birth of a child necessarily implies the renewal of connections to the parent's own narcissism (Freud 1914), the foundational basis for the establishment of the child's initial movement toward subjectivization. When, however, "narcissistic scenarios" (Manzano, J., Espasa, F. P., and Zilkha, N. [1999]. The narcissistic scenarios of parenthood. *International journal of Psychoanalysis*, 80:465–476) predominate, it is the new-born's subjectivization that pays the price (Cahn 2009).

Topics connected to parenthood allow us to investigate an additional temporality of trauma, a possible new iteration of *Nachträglichkeit:* what is transmitted over generations in the complex interplay of identifications, projections, and counter identifications that characterize the parent–new-born relationship (Manzano et al. 1999; Faimberg 1993, 2005b).

This temporality will also be analysed through an examination of the role of the object in constructing the ego and its functioning through the complex system of identifications and projections that connects the passage of psychic life between generations (Kaës et al. 1993). This is an area of investigation that over time has had important developments, among which is Abraham and Torok's concept of the "crypt" (1978). This concept defines the way in which the child's psychic world incorporates deposits of psychic material originating in the parents – a "telescoping" between the generations, a term with which Faimberg (2005b) describes the narcissistic modality and the unconscious identifications in which three generations are condensed.

Within this perspective, as we will see in greater detail in the chapter on parent-child psychotherapies, there have been important applications to child and adolescent analysis as well, starting from the pioneering work of Selma Fraiberg et al. (Fraiberg et al. 1975) on ghosts in the nursery. This was followed in particular by the Geneva School with the first works by Cramer (1974) and Cramer and Palacio Espasa (1993) on brief parent-child interventions, up to the aforementioned survey on the narcissistic settings of parenthood by Manzano et al. (1999).

Relational Dimensions of Trauma Brought to Light in the Analytic Consulting Room

"Doctor, has the door changed? Is something different?" asks Angela with growing unease. In her third year of analysis, she reacts with intense anxiety to the fact that, after exhaustive discussions, the governing board of the condominium building where my office is located has decided to replace the old door, made of ugly yellow aluminium, with a new, more elegant entry door. None of my other patients noticed the change, or at least they had refrained from talking to me about it; Angela, by contrast, urgently needed a reply, needed to feel that her perception was confirmed in my mind.

In the course of her analysis, Angela had been able to put into words her own experiences and to find an interlocutor for the repeated episodes of physical and mental abuse that she had suffered as a child, whose importance had not been grasped by those around her. In this session, Angela brings into the analytic office the dissonance between her memory of what her senses perceived in the past and what she perceives now, reproducing in the transference a disorientation that, some time ago, she had felt but had not been able to share. This feeling was not as connected to the intensity of traumatic excitement to which she was exposed as it was to the relationship with her parents who had not been able to support her in her development.

This brief clinical vignette about a case that will be taken up more extensively later on allows us to deepen our reflections on trauma, especially with respect to its effects in determining identificatory structures and thought processes and with respect to the *basic fault* (Balint 2013), a consequence of a failure to bond with the maternal object.

Ferenczi (1934) affirmed that trauma, more than a reaction to elements that cannot be quantitatively coped with, owes its origin to a lack on the part of the adult to support the child's search for meaning. The adult's denial, silence, and negation about the child's experience could give rise to areas of splitting, unintegrated ones, both in affects and in thought processes.

Along the same lines, Balint (1969) asked what makes the experience of abuse traumatic – whether it is the emotional upheaval itself or rather the expropriation of the meaning of the experience on the part of an adult. In describing the genesis of traumatic experience, he emphasized the fundamental role of the object – that is, of the person who fulfils parental functions – in confirming or negating the child's perceptions of the experience, thus risking their confinement to a particular area of the mind, a private and dissociated one.

It is in contexts similar to the early relationship that conditions are created for obstacles to arise in the genesis of the thinking apparatus (Bion 1962b) or for those situations that Winnicott described as characterized by *fear of breakdown* (1974), in which the person who could not feel painful affects tied to a traumatic experience holds within himself the traces of that unlived pain. As Giaconia and Racalbuto (1997) hypothesize, what can be considered traumatic are precisely those events that are not susceptible to representational, psychic working through – those external or internal events that cannot be integrated into psychic reality. Or, as César and Sara Botella (2004) state, the traumatic character cannot derive in every case from the content of an event representable in itself but rather from a mental disorganization that would have its origin in the lack of meaning for an ego still in its formative phases, an ego that could not count on having the mental competence to form mental representations of what was happening.

Angela

Intense suffering and the need to bring some order to her life had led Angela, a woman in her forties, to consult me. She had been through 20 years of a marriage that was now nearly over. She suffered from impoverished communication with her husband, and she defined her life as characterized by "a sense of failure and defeat." What especially worried her was the difficult relationship with her nine-year-old son, who in her opinion "ran along the tracks of a story already written." With these words she was referring to relationships with other important men in her life, in which she inevitably ended up finding herself in a passive situation of subjugation; her relationships had a masochistic tone in which any type of suffering was, in the end, preferable to the experience of being left alone.

Angela suffered from anxiety attacks and periods of depression, among which was an especially dark one after the birth of her son. At that time she had felt a deep sadness accompanied by the feeling, in looking at her own child, of being with a stranger.

From the beginning of the analysis, countertransferential sensations made me feel like a powerful and idealized person who would be able to use her for his own satisfaction, as long as my knowledge "penetrated" her confusion and thus caused her to exit from a state of very intense pain. In our early face-to-face sessions, before moving to the couch, Angela kept her eyes lowered, and only over time did she consent to fleetingly meet my gaze. She communicated a feeling that she was gradually loosening up, and she caused me to think that sensorial aspects of my countertransference were reactivated by the projective identifications of a child who had felt scrutinized by direct stares that focused on her unpleasantness and unworthiness.

The intensity of suffering expressed by Angela was so strong that I noticed the weight of it even after our work together. Returning home from one of our sessions, I had the sensation of having had to leave things in a solidified state, as though the quantity of unelaborated feelings that were directly transmitted in all their intensity required a sort of psychic digestion on my part as well.

Angela had been born into a family of a patriarchal cast, in which both men and women were dedicated to work and subjugated their own needs to the timing and necessities of the family's artisanal business. It was a family about which one might hypothesize disappointment at the birth of a girl instead of a boy.

In what appeared to be a sea of extreme deprivation and acute family conflicts, similar to what one might find in a fairy tale set in olden times, the positive figure of a grandmother emerged – a woman who, when the level of family conflict got too high, took Angela with her into her room, where they passed the time telling each other stories.

Angela had an older sister and brother who left home early on. She, in contrast, stayed behind. As soon as it was possible, however, Angela became engaged to a man of about the same age as she, who quickly revealed himself to be overbearing and violent. His abusive behaviours seemed to her to be the price to pay in order to stay with him. Their sexual relationship, which she had imagined as very romantic, in reality had been imposed on her and proved disappointing; she did not feel pleasure but pretended to do so in order to satisfy her fiancé, as she did with the other men in her life, tolerating the problem as a further expression of her own unworthiness.

Sexuality appeared to be a great enigma in Angela's life, one toward which she felt an interest but at the same time a sense of repulsion and shame. These feelings were expressed in the transference, as on the occasion of a dream in which she found herself in bed looking up at a hanging lamp that was swinging in an earthquake. Nearby there was a man who, when she asked him to reassure her and give her a hug, told her that she would have to cope with the earthquake on her own. In fact, Angela had the impression that everyone had always told her she would have to cope on her own, and she would have been ready for anything if she were not told to cope on her own by me as well.

In the course of the analysis, memories emerged of childhood sexual activities that were never joyful. She marvelled at her own impression of having holes in her memory; she couldn't manage to come up with an exact recollection of these activities, events that she "didn't have in mind." They ranged from excessive exposure to a sexual scene between two adults, to sexual games that were desired but also undergone as the price to pay in order to be accepted – to the point of actual abuse.

Angela related:

> I don't have a precise memory of what I did with my friends; I know that there are some things I don't have in mind. I was among the smallest ones in a group of neighborhood children. I remember "that" room in a friend's house – not an exact memory, but at first I was considered a foolish little girl, someone to play tricks on, and then something changed. I became part of a group, and meanwhile "these things" happened. It wasn't a kind of play in which we were all on equal footing [she commented, starting to cry] – they didn't force me, it was like entering into something and becoming part of it and not being alone; it was a strange game of intimacy. I was too little. There was nothing exciting about all this, but afterward I felt I began to be taken seriously. And paradoxically, I have the memory of a smell, the smell of one of those boys mixed with the smell of that room. For years I carried the idea inside that sexuality was a way to be recognized, and this allowed me to overcome anything.

Little by little, other episodes of violence emerged, part of a childhood characterized by few specific memories, as though wrapped in a fog. In one of these, a man who did sales and marketing for the family business touched her breast, and this gave her a sense of disgust. Nonetheless, she remembered that, to some degree, she liked interacting with this man because she felt she had his attention. On one occasion she had tried to speak of it with her mother, but her account was not taken seriously.

Angela continued to feel that a piece of her life was "missing"; she felt she could think about herself as a child and would then suddenly shift to imagining herself as an adult. She had no memories of her adolescence; she seemed to have suddenly become older without there being a basis for maturity, and it was hard for her to imagine what her son would be like at that age.

Angela's question "Can it be that a person eliminates something from her story or may have only fragments of something that happened?" united her with Ivan's mother and others who had had to face the reality of abuse and who later lived an experience of fragmentation and dissociation.

Giorgio

While she was pregnant, Angela had had a feeling of total well-being for the only time in her life; she described the feeling as "fullness." During the gestational period, oedipal fantasies were evident in her attunement with herself, from the moment that her father showed joy and interest in her pregnancy. She felt highly thought of, valued as her brother was, as though she possessed the penis that she had felt to be missing, her father's penis inside herself. The feeling of fullness and happiness was connected to the narcissistic reflection and social recognition of oedipal fantasies; it immediately disappeared after she gave birth.

With the arrival of her son, Angela felt abandoned by everyone. No longer did she have a big belly; instead she had before her a stranger. The strangeness of her son, so different from what she had imagined, created a new place for a reality that was very familiar to her: the way he looked at her and seemed not to trust her reminded her of the way that her husband, brother, and father looked at her. Giorgio was a difficult baby with very disturbed sleep from the day he was born.

The analysis allowed Angela to question herself about how her son fit into the line-up of males in her life who surrounded her. It was as though Giorgio was "wearing clothes that didn't belong to him," having been assigned to the role of one of the many abusive characters in her internal world that was permeated by trauma and violence.

Angela vacillated between attempts to position herself as a mother who helped her son grow up as different from herself and the experiences of a little girl who felt violated by a male whom she could not oppose without fear of losing him and being abandoned. She had the impression that the baby was an issue that pertained only to her – not to her husband and herself as a couple – and that the responsibility for the baby's behaviour fell exclusively onto her. Oedipal guilt again arose, with its need for expiation after the brief "honeymoon" of pregnancy, and this guilt mixed with the sense of narcissistic failure that she felt in the face of the otherness of her son, who presented as hostile to her. Her husband, for his part, did not seem capable of achieving the developmental passage from companion to parent, and, in a kind of generalized jealousy, he blamed her and verbally threatened her and the child when the child cried, attributing to Angela the responsibility for everything that didn't go well.

Manzano et al. (1999) affirm that often some parents relive through their children the rage that they felt toward their own parents, counter-identifying with the hated parent in a masochistic way. In these situations, it isn't possible to set limits on the children's wishes for fear of unleashing uncontainable aggression. Angela had always felt that her mom was "bad" and had promised herself that she would not become like her. And so she was patient, not reacting or reacting only by trying to persuade her son with words. In the end she "pardoned" him as she had "pardoned" her father, her brother, and later her husband, thinking that, overall, it was normal that they should treat her that way. Over the course of the analysis, parallels between her son, her brother, and her husband – all aggressive and abusive toward Angela – emerged with ever greater force.

There was an attempt through sexuality to come to a resolution of what had been missing from the patient's life. Abraham (1907) spoke of child abuse as a sexual theory; Angela's childhood sexual theory was that sexuality had narcissistic value, which led her to desire a sexuality in which she had to be at the beck and call of others in order to be accepted.

Haydee Faimberg (2005b, pp. 75–76) connected "a certain narcissistic functioning to an oedipal context," speaking of the "o-o" logic, a narcissistic dimension of the oedipal conflict that is reactivated in the transference. In the narcissistic object relation, the child represents the ego ideal of the parents, and in some cases he must receive from them not only what the parents received in the past but also, especially, what they most missed (ibid., p. 81).

During the course of an analysis, identifying an excessive narcissistic dimension in the parent-child relationship is an important moment at which to be able to resolve the processes of projective identification that bind the child to the role of an important character in the parents' story. Angela recounted:

> My son put me in embarrassing situations. He would be deliberately rude, to the point that at times others would intervene when I should have been the one to do so. Sometimes I had the impression that my son wanted to punish me for something, and in those situations I didn't know what to do.

Manzano et al. (1999) listed four basic elements present in "parental narcissistic scenarios": a projection of the parents onto the child; the parents' complementary identification (counter-identification); a specific objective; and dynamic relational acting out. In these authors' opinion, a parent's projection onto a child constitutes a projective identification, which in all cases involves the accomplishment of narcissistic satisfaction. Repetition of the trauma represents an attempt to counteract psychic collapse, and the acted-out interaction is the result of these projections and identifications, which happen in reality; they influence relationships and go beyond the imaginary.

At times, internal images are projected into the child, images that are "pregnant with aggression and destruction" (Manzano et al. 1999, p. 113, translation by G. Atkinson). The parent feels persecuted by a child who is the carrier of projections of his or her own characteristics, which coexist with libidinal ties that successfully maintain the connection. Sometimes incestuous and abusive objects are projected. In the couple, there is no transition from a two-way dimension to a three-way one, which would complete the mourning process stemming from the desire to be the child of one's partner; in these situations, the child can become the carrier, at a fantasized level, of a threatening otherness.

Individualizing Elements

Little by little, at times, Angela was able to see her son as a child – different and separate from her and free of the anxieties that had been projected onto him. She related that her son, too, seemed to marvel at finding himself with a different sort of mom, one who located herself in relation to him as a separate person and who did not directly compare him to other men in the family.

Angela found herself wishing that her son would stay little, not only to allow her to feel affection and tenderness toward him – feelings that in her family of origin were considered awkward – but also almost as though to slow down the emergence of an aggressive and abusive sexuality that seemed to be casting a pall over his development. Fears about her son's coming adolescence led her to consider her own as well: "At times it seems to me that a piece of my life is missing, and I would like to understand whether I, too, was ever really a teenager."

In the course of our sessions, Angela began to remember episodes from her childhood that stirred up intense pain. In one of these, she had marked out a small space in the yard in which to create a little garden; she had put a little fence around it and placed her dolls inside. The border, the garden, and the dolls were all swept away in a single action by her father, who did not tolerate "silliness of this kind." In the same way, her internal borders had been violated by her mother, who on finding Angela's diary – in which she had written something intimate – had ripped it up.

The theme of a private space that she couldn't permit herself to have had been expressed from the beginning in relation to the analysis as well; to be able to make use of a psychic and temporal space exposed her to criticism from the masculine characters in her internal world: "it costs too much" and "you're neglecting your family" were the most common criticisms. At the same time, a transference of a masochistic/undifferentiated type continued to unfold, in line with which – in a state in which she was only barely psychically differentiated from me – she would have accepted paying any price as long as I, who had the possibility of doing so, kept her close.

After some years of analysis, Angela revealed that she felt very guilty about a dream she had had:

> There is a party in a room; there are some balloons floating in the air, and my son is sitting on top of one of the balloons. I help him to get off, but at a certain point I notice that both he and the balloon have vanished, have gone out through a skylight. I am seized by great anxiety at the thought that my son might be dead, and I suddenly wake up.

In this dream, in which there seems to be a distinction between the representation of the patient's self and the representation of her son, Angela met with a separation that activated death anxieties. The flow of associations led her to say:

> Do you know that when my son was born, I didn't want him? I was doing so well while I was pregnant, and then everyone started demanding things of me – the baby cried, my milk didn't come in, and everyone said it was my fault, they blamed me when he cried. Then my son became something for which I was responsible; I had to mediate between him and the world, and it was as though we were only a single thing.

Angela felt guilty when she assumed any autonomous position. In what I imagined as a collateral transference – a transference shifted onto someone who is not the analyst – she had a relationship with the first man with whom she had felt free. For the first time she experienced an orgasm, and she felt herself to be a "normal" woman, without having to pay for it with a sexuality that depended on her being accepted by a man.

Over time she had begun to let herself start to imagine how much she would have liked to have a different relationship with Giorgio. She noticed herself experiencing many states of mind as also mirrored in her son: "I don't know if there is a sort of symbiosis or if I am merely relieving many of my things through him." Now and then, Angela managed to see her son as another person, with an autonomy that she herself had never had, and she liked to imagine him as different from herself and from the men in her life.

Elements of Reconciliation – The Present Rewrites the Past

In the course of our sessions, the potential for a possible reconciliation with her father had begun to take shape, placing him within the limits of a familial, working-class environment in which a certain lack of feeling was necessary in order to ensure survival in the market in that atmosphere, which she described as one of extreme rigidity and gratuitous mental violence.

Regarding her relationship with her ex-husband – though with some degree of jealousy because of the positive relationship that their son was establishing with him – she managed to find some positive factors for the child there and to hypothesize a more definitive separation from her ex-husband. She imagined a move to a new home or simply not allowing him to visit her.

In this recovery of a distinct and subjective dimension of her own, Angela began to be able to set limits on her son's behaviour and, with surprise, she noticed that if she succeeded in staying firm when he became overbearing the explosions of rage that she had feared didn't happen. Indeed, Giorgio seemed reassured and, in a short time, he could resume their relationship. Being able to see her own aggression without feeling herself to be as destructive as she had feared allowed Angela to understand the need for limits that her son required and led her to say: "He wants me to be the mom."

She also began to experience greater closeness in her relationship with her own mother. Angela remembered that, on one occasion, her mother had talked to her about a relative who had suffered from serious depression and had added that if this relative had gotten treatment earlier, she might have led a very different life. This memory led Angela to think of what she herself was doing and to derive satisfaction from it. She noticed, almost with astonishment, the pleasure that she felt in having refound this positive relationship and in rethinking the occasion when she had once said to herself that she would not like to be like her mother. She told herself that her real meaning had been that she would not have wanted to have all those regrets or to lose the relationship with her own children.

In the transference, maternal fantasies also emerged, and these allowed Angela to "place" her mother in a different position: "It is nice to have found my mom!" That also permitted her to be fully aware of how much she had tried, with her own son, to establish a relationship diametrically opposed to the one she had had with her mother. Cramer (1974; Cramer and Palacio Espasa 1993) would say that Angela identified both with the angry child who she herself had been and masochistically with her hated mother. Here, however, the picture got more complicated because both vertices of the parental couple were problematic, and in the background there was guilt about the desire to have a baby from an aggressive father, seen as the only way to be accepted as a person.

In situations like this, I often find myself thinking of primary narcissism nourished by the loving gaze that the mother directs to her child's body, in this way transmitting to him her own narcissism and that of the father. And of how it happens that, on this basis, the child constructs his own feeling of existence, his first love for himself.

Toward the Conclusion of the Analysis

During the period in which she was in analysis, Angela's relationship with her son markedly improved, and she was able to release him from the projective identifications that compared him to other men in her life and, in the transference, to the analyst. The relationship with her mother, too, was modified, and now she felt close to her; at times she was sorry for not having been able to give her mother more. Angela succeeded in distinguishing the father of her childhood and adolescence from her father of today, who was coping with the final stages of his life.

> At times I feel divided in two – the father who, when he was sick, greeted me by giving me a kiss is not compatible with the one who, now cured, sends me away. Do you know that I no longer have bad dreams? No more do I have those dreams with an erotic backdrop where "these" men left me. The negative quality of those dreams was almost an obsession, and I felt shameless; there was no violence, but there was abandonment, derision, someone who seemed to say to me: "It was all a joke, and you fell for it again." I feel more comfortable at home now because I've found myself again, and when one finds oneself, everything is easier. It also happened that I allowed myself to have sex with someone I've known for a while. I asked myself for a long time if I would be capable of having sex in a detached way, and now I don't even pose the question. I had sex, there was no great sentimental involvement, and I sort of liked it and sort of didn't – but it wasn't something that made me anxious.

In the face of what could have been a collateral transference in a relational system dominated by the "confusion of tongues" (Ferenczi 1932) – in which, for Angela, sex had been a misleading way of not feeling the experience of humiliation and abandonment – I was thinking about the fact that we were at the third to the last session before our agreed-upon ending date of the analysis. I pointed out to Angela that she was now able to think that our relationship would end without necessarily having to feel abandoned and mocked – that she wouldn't have to do anything to avoid abandonment, that there was a difference between the sexual dimension and that of relationships. She said:

> I don't feel like the same person any more. Before, I kept everything inside and I seemed to be saying, "Do to me what you will." Now this happens much less, even though I still feel the strain of setting limits.
>
> I've made peace with men, with males – maybe I've become a little more clever, more clear. The difference is that now things hit me less hard. In her final years of life, my grandmother wasn't well; I slept with her and I knew how to manage her – when she was agitated, I took her hand and calmed her down.

It seems that now Angela has taken back those qualities of caregiving that allow her to take care of her confused, agitated, violated parts. She can also accept the end of the analysis, highlighting precisely the backward direction of *Nachträglichkeit* in the psychoanalytic experience, which allows for a retranscription of past experiences and their retroactive revision.

The work done by Angela led to positive changes in her son as well, at least in the internal son who was called up in the sessions. The psychic work of the mother to rid herself of idiosyncratic projections liberated him from an emotional weight that did not permit him to find his own individual and subjective place in the generational order, releasing – in a way that one might imagine to be long-lasting – the temporal expressions of trauma as well, which would potentially be capable of influencing subsequent generations.

Note

1   See Laplanche and Pontalis 1973; Thomä and Cheshire 1991; Laplanche 1998; Ferraro and Garella 2009; Eickhoff 2008; Faimberg 2005a; Birksted-Breen 2003; Parsons 2009; Marion 2012.

References

Abraham, K. (1907). The experiencing of sexual traumas as a form of sexual activity. In *Selected Papers of Karl Abraham*. New York: Brunner/Mazel, 1979, pp. 47–63.

Abraham, N. & Torok, M. (1978). *The Shell and the Kernel*, ed. & trans. N. T. Rand. Chicago, IL/London: University of Chicago Press, 1994.

Balint, M. (1969). Trauma and object relationship. *Int. J. Psychoanal.*, 50:429–435.

———. (2013). *The Basic Fault: Therapeutic Aspects of Regression*. London: Routledge.

Baranger, W., Baranger, M. & Mom, J. (1988). The infantile psychic trauma from us to Freud: Pure trauma, retroactivity, and reconstruction. *Int. J. Psychoanal.*, 69:113–128.

Bion, W. R. (1962b). *Learning from Experience*. London: Routledge, 1984.

Birksted-Breen, D. (2003). Time and the *après-coup. Int. J. Psychoanal.*, 84:1501–1515.

Bokanowski, T. (2005). Variations on the concept of traumatism: Traumatism, traumatic, trauma. *Int. J. Psychoanal.*, 86:251–265.

Botella, C. & Botella, S. (2004). *The Work of Psychic Figurability: Mental States without Representation*, trans. A. Weller. London: New Library of Psychoanalysis.

Cahn, R. (2009). Una vita di lavoro con gli adolescenti [A life working with adolescents]. In "Essere Adolescenti oggi" ["Being Adolescents Today"], ed. R. Goisis & S. Bonfiglio. *I quaderni del Centro Milanese di Psicoanalisi [Notes from the Milanese Psychoanalytic Center]*, Milano: Quaderni del Centro Milanese di Psicoanalisi.

Cramer, B. (1974). Interventions thérapeutiques brèves avec parents et enfantas. *Psychiatrie de l'enfant*, 17:53–117.

Cramer, B. & Palacio Espasa, F. (1993). *Le psicoterapie madre bambino*. Milano: Masson, 1995.

Dahl, G. (2010). The two-time vectors of *Nachträglichkeit* in the development of ego organization: Significance of the concept for the symbolization of nameless traumas and anxieties. *Int. J. Psychoanal.*, 91:727–744.

Eickhoff, F. W. (2008). Sulla *Nachträglichkeit*: la modernità di un vecchio concetto [On *Nachträglichkeit*: The modernity of an old concept]. *L'Annata Psicoanalitica*, 4:129–144.

Faimberg, H. (1993). All'ascolto del télescopage delle generazioni: pertinenza psicoanalitica del concetto [Listening to the telescoping of generations: Psychoanalytic relevance of the concept]. In *Trasmissione della vita psichica tra le generazioni [Transmission of Psychic Life Between Generations]*, ed. R. Kaës, H. Faimberg, M. Enriquez & J. J. Baranez. Roma: Borla, 1995.

———. (2005a). Après-coup. *Int. J. Psychoanal.*, 86:1–6.

———. (2005b). *The Telescoping of Generations: Listening to the Narcissistic Links Between Generations*. London: New Library of Psychoanalysis.

Ferenczi, S. (1932). The confusion of tongues between adults and the child: The language of tenderness and passion. In *Final Contributions to the Problems and Methods of Psycho-Analysis*, ed. M. Balint. New York: Brunner/Mazel, 1980, pp. 156–167.

———. (1934). *Reflections on Trauma the Psychoanalytic Review (1913–1957)* (Vol. 25). New York.

Ferraro, F. & Garella, A. (2009). *Nachträglichkeit*. In *Forme dell'après-coup [Forms of Après-Coup]*, ed. M. Balsamo. Milano: FrancoAngeli.

Fraiberg, S., Adelson, E. & Shapiro, V. (1975). Ghosts in the nursery: A psychoanalytic approach to the problems of impaired infant-mother relationships. *J. Amer. Acad. Child & Adolescent Psychiatry*, 14:387–421.

Freud, A. (1936). *The Ego and the Mechanisms of Defense*. London: Karnac, 1993.

———. (1895). Project for a scientific psychology. *S. E.*, 1.

———. (1896). Further remarks on the neuro-psychoses of defence. *S. E.*, 3

———. (1914). On narcissism: An introduction. *S. E.*, 14.

———. (1915). Mourning and melancholia. *S. E.*, 14.

———. (1917). Introductory lectures on psycho-analysis. *S. E.*, 15–16.

———. (1918). From the history of an infantile neurosis (the "Wolf Man"). *S. E.*, 17.

———. (1925). Some psychical consequences of the anatomical distinction between the sexes. *S. E.*, 19.

———. (1935). Inhibitions, symptoms and anxiety. *Psychoanal. Q.*, 4:616–625.

———. (1937a). Analysis terminable and interminable. *S. E.*, 23.

———. (1937b). Constructions in analysis. *S. E.*, 23.

———. (1934–1938). Moses and monotheism. *S. E.*, 23.

Giaconia, G. & Racalbuto, A. (1997). Il circolo vizioso trauma-fantasma-trauma [The vicious cycle of trauma-fantasm-trauma]. *Rivista di Psicoanalisi*, 43:541–558.

Kaës, R., Faimberg, H., Enriquez, M. & Baranes, J. J. (1993). *Trasmissione della vita psichica tra le generazioni [Transmission of Psychic Life Between Generations]*. Roma: Borla, 1995.

Laplanche, J. (1987). *New Foundations for Psychoanalysis*, trans. D. Macey. Cambridge, MA/Oxford, UK: Basil Blackwell, 1989.

Laplanche, J. & Pontalis, J.-B. (1973). *The Language of Psycho-Analysis*, trans. D. Nicholson-Smith. London: Hogarth.

Manzano, J., Espasa, F. P. & Zilkha, N. (1999). The narcissistic scenarios of parenthood. *Int. J. Psychoanal.*, 80:465–476.

Marion, P. (2012). Some reflections on the unique time of *Nachträglichkeit* in theory and clinical practice. *Int. J. Psychoanal.*, 93:317–340.

Parsons, M. (2009). Après-coup and Avant coup: Death and the primal scene. *European Psa. Federation Bull.*, 63:150–157.

Thomä, H. & Cheshire, N. (1991). Freud's *Nachträglichkeit* and Strachey's "deferred action": Trauma, constructions, and the direction of causality. *Int. J. Psychoanal.*, 18:407–427.

Turo, J. (2013). Resuscitation of the concept of *Nachträglichkeit:* Its role in psychoanalytic process and therapeutic action. Paper presented at IPA Congress, Prague.

Winnicott, D. W. (1974). Fear of breakdown. *Int. Rev. Psychoanal.*, 1:103–107.

Chapter 4

Communicating the Diagnosis

The Fine Line Between Pain and Trauma

Maria was 12 years old, and for a month she had been in hospitals. Brought to a session because she wasn't growing much, a doctor in a facility in the city where she lived had hypothesized the possible presence of a genetic condition that, with substantially normal psychic and cognitive development, involved stunted physical growth and some problems in the area of gynaecology and with sterility. That had caused Maria's mother to go into a deep depression, and at first it had made her reject the diagnosis that had been confirmed a month later by the centre where I practiced.

When I met the girl, she had been taken in for definitive testing some days earlier. She had not been told anything about her situation, and apparently she had asked nothing. I had met the parents on a Friday morning, and they were by now resigned; they appeared oppressed by an enormous weight that seemed to have hardened the father's personality and crushed the mother by a pain that was constantly at risk of being expressed in sobs, which were held back only with difficulty.

They didn't know what to tell their daughter about something that they didn't know how to talk about to themselves, and the idea didn't occur to them that Maria had formed some hypotheses herself about what was happening. It wasn't a problem to them that a bright and intelligent 12-year-old – who had been brought to the hospital for every sort of exam and who in one month had seen her mother become sad, immersed in a dark mood, while she accompanied her to a long sequence of exams, lab tests, and x-rays – might have needed to come up with an idea about what was happening, to have some explanations, and if this didn't happen, she had probably concluded it was something very serious.

When I called this to the parents' attention, they had essentially agreed that it seemed strange to them as well that an intelligent girl like their daughter, otherwise so curious, now exhibited a complete lack of curiosity and cooperated in a docile way with whatever her parents proposed to her.

In the course of our meeting, the parents were essentially persuaded that it could be useful to Maria to have something explained to her, to give her a sense of all that was happening, but they did not feel able to do this. They asked, though

DOI: 10.4324/9781003252238-5

quite apprehensively, to be helped with that by a specialist with whom they would meet that afternoon, together with Maria.

In that much-awaited meeting, the doctor had explained what the clinical situation consisted of, in its auxologic, endocrine implications and also the difficulties that could occur for Maria in the future if she were to carry a pregnancy to term naturally. The girl had listened and had asked all the questions that she felt were necessary, and once she had the answers, she had posed the main question: "But is this everything? There's nothing else?" – allowing it to be understood that her greatest fear related to the possible presence of an incurable illness.

If on the one hand the idea of an incurable illness, in the child's fantasies, could be the idea of an illness with an unfavourable prognosis; at an emotional level, there was a risk of her thinking her condition was not curable because it could not even be expressed.

Communicating and Not Communicating

Communicating a diagnosis represents a difficult operation, especially when it gives a name to something that can undermine well-being or indeed risk a person's life. Today it takes on a disquieting immediacy when new medical and scientific technologies, such as current genetic molecular research investigations, allow us to confront somatic territories that were unthinkable up to a short time ago. These pose new problems regarding the emotional impact on the patient and his family.

Resorting to a hospital is often linked to a discrete fact, and even when there is a recovery connected to pathologies with benign prognoses, an emotional event with traumatic potentiality always hovers in the background. The way in which things come to be spoken about – that is, how diagnoses are communicated – is very important at a time when the patient and his family are in a state of deep distress, which can momentarily give them the impression of not being capable, either emotionally or at a concrete level, of mustering the skills that the new situation demands.

In the situations under discussion, one often has to deal with people who suddenly find themselves facing an event that, from one moment to the next, has transformed normal everyday life into a torturous journey that leads them to encounter new surroundings, with new rules that they don't know, with a logical framework and habits that are different from the usual ones, and with a heavy and threatening shadow, the illness, that suddenly seems to cast doubt on the prospects and indeed the possibility of a future life.

So this is not about transmitting cognitive contents; the knowledge that must be transmitted is inexorably interwoven with intense emotions tied to deep anxieties of existence. Often, pain is such that psychological defence mechanisms are activated, ones that do not allow the person to understand or to hold in memory what is said to them. A paediatrician who, at the end of a long day of work, had dedicated two hours to explaining to a parent the pathology his child was suffering from could not understand the fact that, the next day, not even a trace remained of what he had tried to say the day before.

Communicating a diagnosis requires time; it doesn't happen on the spot in a single action but through a process of communication between the patient and his family, the treating clinician and his group of colleagues: the doctors, nurses, and national health insurance workers in charge of the situation. How often does it happen that the most productive communications, the actual moments of emotional and cognitive integration, take place at informal moments – such as during night-time hours, when beyond the established procedures, a parent turns to a nurse who can help him give an understandable form to the totality of information that, during the daytime, his mind has not managed to integrate?

In fact, it is necessary to leave space for the work of mourning, that is, the process of emotional working through that the subject must accomplish to overcome the psychic pain caused by a loss – for example, loss of the state of health that he has known – and to re-establish and reorganize a new psychic balance.

The work of mourning has its well-known internal oppositional forces: first, shock and rebellion, then anger, then a depressive condition that can slide down into melancholy – that is, the affective state connected to an unworked-through loss to which the subject attributes responsibility (Freud 1915).

In these delicate situations, when the emotional balance both within the individual and in the family is shaken by the encounter with pathology, the level of suffering is so intense that it is necessary to devote time to its working through. Only with time can one actually arrive at a different balance and limit the recourse to psychological self-protective mechanisms, which entail the risk that unthought and unworked-through areas will remain active in the patient's mind and the minds of his family members. Often the intensity of suffering is maintained intact, as though emotional life freezes, arrested at the zero hour represented by the appearance of the diagnosis of illness.

In the field of paediatrics, communicating the diagnosis is something that involves the doctor, the parents, and the child – to whom, via the parent and the doctor, the diagnosis must be told.

The consequences of communicating a diagnosis, in the situation of a child's pathology, have similar characteristics to those seen in trauma, and, like all traumatic experiences, these consequences have the capacity to throw into crisis established balances, to reactivate primitive emotional situations present in every individual at the deepest mental levels.

The reactions to these events are affected by the extent of the problem, by the capacity for resilience, by the patient's previous experiences and those of his family, and by the way in which the situation comes to be presented and followed by the group of caregivers.

Communicating the diagnosis represents one of those "impossible tasks" for which the right solutions are very difficult to identify and seem to run along a fine line that divides a painful experience from a traumatic one, with the implied risk of veering to one side or the other. Psychic pain can be considered a discrepancy between the internal representation that a person ideally has of himself and the representation that he has of the current state of the self, in both somatic terms and in psychological ones (Joffe and Sandler 1965). Pain can encourage motivational or adaptive forces that can modify the situation and propose new balances.

To summarize what was described in a previous chapter, from an emotional point of view, trauma refers to tensions in excess of what the psychic apparatus can sustain. It isn't so much that contents can be traumatic; more often, it is the impossibility of having a psychic transcription of the trauma so that it can be transformed into mental contents. The essence of trauma is that of an excess of emotions relative to the possibility of accomplishing this function of psychic transformation.

Antonino Ferro maintains that mental suffering can be primarily due to two kinds of factors – one stemming mainly from missing environmental elements and the other from the child's constitutional fragility in withstanding tension and in elaborating his emotions. To these he adds situations in which

> the quantity of sensory stimulation, whether exteroceptive or proprioceptive, outstrips the capacity of the alpha function to form alpha elements. We then have a "traumatic" situation, in which the quantitative level of stimulation (beta elements) exceeds what can be transformed into alpha and rendered thinkable.
>
> [Ferro 2002, p. 2]

A Sufficiently Solid Container

An eight-year-old child with some psychological problems, in addition to a physical problem, was used to engaging in artistic activity in her sessions with me. She did it in a very creative way, expressing with her designs the emotional difficulties that she had to confront. During two sessions, she used sheets of paper to construct shapes. At the first of these sessions, she had begun to make big envelopes that contained smaller envelopes, which in turn contained even smaller ones, to the point that, in the end, a very small envelope contained a very small piece of paper with a sort of secret puzzle.

In that session, she had not told me what the problem was that needed to be resolved, but at the next one, she constructed a durable box made of paper, strengthened by corners made of little pieces of modelling clay.

After the child had worked a while in silence, I saw her cheer up when I asked her if by chance the need to construct a kind of container allowed her to express her concern that we couldn't keep between ourselves the thoughts that she wasn't sure of being able to express to me. In other words, did the construction of containers convey her fear that I was not a sufficiently solid container for her?

Ferro's categorization proposes a brief new immersion in the thinking of Wilfred Bion, who provided us with especially useful elements with which to understand early emotions that are represented or reactivated under particular circumstances.

Thanks to the maternal function that Bion called "reverie," which we have already encountered in previous chapters, the child is helped to improve his internal reality and to transform it into figurable and representable elements. In time he finds the way to make this capacity his and to exercise it on his own.

That calls directly into play the function of listening and acceptance, which constitutes a characteristic of interpersonal relationships and plays a specific role in the caregiving professions.

Elements of this type are at play when we live the experience of listening – when we hear that a parent is bringing us something worrisome that, for him, is not amenable to mental working through, and after our meeting he goes away with a different facial expression. We don't really know what we have done, but it is possible that we have listened to his concerns with an emotional attitude of listening and that even having merely held his worries in our mind may play a part in filtering out their disquieting aspects.

In effect, knowledge about the state of illness and the emotional states associated with it is often feared as overly intense. Many times some parents hesitate to allow a child to participate in a diagnosis that pertains to him, with the result that a state of not telling, not communicating, is created – which, as in Maria's case, leads the child to fear a diagnosis much worse than the real one. This is because, fully perceiving what is happening around him, the child begins to feel that it is something that cannot even be talked about.

In many situations, communicating the diagnosis comes as a liberation for the child, who with relief learns in an intelligible way something that he had noticed in its intensity but that he hadn't been able to translate into thought.

If the child needs to be protected from overly intense experiences, at the same time, he also has an inalienable right to be recognized in his capacity to understand what is happening to him.

In the context of a family's emotional climate that has been decisively altered and is different from what it was prior to contact with the hospital, when the child turns to another adult to understand and give meaning to what he has experienced, he may receive from this adult – who cannot tolerate the pain that the child's needs cause to resound in him – a non-answer or a denial. In the discrepancy between what the senses perceive on the one hand and the words that do not explain what happened on the other, it is the capacity to think that ends up being inhibited. This second time of trauma consists in blocking the child from finding the meaning of what has happened to him, from being able to translate it into words, from thinking it and having a mental representation of it.

I think that, even in a place dedicated to acute illnesses – most notably the hospital – it is important to offer the parents the possibility of not being isolated by and submersed under the weight of emotions that are so difficult to bear.

Usually, the medical and health personnel who work alongside parents who are having difficulties help them bolster their adult parts and their competence in caring for their children. At certain moments, the parents may seem threatened by feelings of incapacity, inadequacy, and impotence. The aim is to recover the skills that, according to Harris and Meltzer (2013), underlie the parental function: to help children contain depressive pain and keep alive in them their hope, love, and thinking.

At the age of five-and-a-half years, Francesca was diagnosed with a rather rare endocrine disorder. Her parents had consulted doctors in the area where she had grown up; these physicians knew very little about the disorder. They had told the parents that this was a very serious illness but without being able either to administer an appropriate treatment or to explain exactly what the disorder consisted of. From research on the internet, the parents' fears had gradually increased, and for two or three years they had worried that this was a tumorous disorder with an unfortunate prognosis over time. After the correct diagnosis was made and a therapy instigated that was then scaled back to periodic check-ups to determine the exact quantity of synthetic hormones to be administered – which would guarantee a good quality of life over time – the parents had not been able to explain to their daughter what had happened to her or what the problem that afflicted her consisted of. The physical pain involved in numerous lab tests and other medical procedures, which were difficult to varying degrees, did not seem to worry Francesca. Instead, her worries seemed to relate to not knowing, to not having the words that would give meaning to what was happening around her. Indeed, she was the centre of interest for many persons – her parents and various specialists; these people all treated her as though at her age she lacked any curiosity, concerns, thoughts, or fantasies about what was happening to her, which they would have been required to take into consideration in finding answers and the means with which to express themselves, according to the resources that children have at their disposal in the various stages of their development.

"I was little but I wasn't a fool," Francesca would say to a caregiver in the course of a session, speaking of her childhood illness and of the many silences that her questions met with.

There is often an assumption of dullness on the part of children, which can make sense only if thought of as an attribution to the child of a bewildered and limited mental state in the parent who has been struck by a pain that is too intense. Here a part of the child that remains separate, traumatized, isolated, and undeveloped coexists alongside parts of the parents, competent and capable of taking care of their children.

There is a widespread tendency to keep children distanced and in the dark about pain and losses that occur in the course of life and not to notice that it is not as important that children avoid suffering as it is that, in those moments, they can find someone to console them and to share their pain.

And when parents come to the hospital, very often they find themselves regressing into a situation of dependence that casts them as frightened children.

In thinking about trauma, we have seen that there is a quantity and a quality of emotions characterized by a "too muchness" relative to the resources of children and parents, which one must be aware of in considering the children and their relationships with health care institutions.

Understanding the potentially traumatic element for the parents of a communication about their son's or daughter's pathology represents a fundamentally important starting point in allowing parents to eventually overcome the traumatic impact.

Some propose communicative techniques that make it possible to give "bad news" in a "good" way. I do not think this is possible; news that shatters the way of life that has supported the child's growth and a parent's ideal self must be taken into consideration in all its explosive intensity.

Bursting into the internal landscape of fantasies that have to do with primary levels of psychic integration, with internal objects that have been irreparably damaged and compromised precisely in the early phases of an individual's fantasy life, brings back irreparable losses that only subsequent developments and acquisitions can keep integrated in a balance that, though stable, is sometimes destabilized by particularly difficult events.

What should we say, however, about pains of the soul when the child's pain does not arrive at an adult who is able to recognize him, understand him, and console him?

Pain in the Parent

Paolo, whose parents are Anna and Luigi, was identified at birth as having an endocrine disorder that would allow him to lead an absolutely normal life but that made it necessary for him to have periodic laboratory tests and hospital stays and to take hormone replacements for the rest of his life. At our first meeting, the parents appeared to be enclosed in their pain, an enclosure connected more to a reserved personality – that of the father – while the mother's personality was more marked by conflict.

Somewhat against their will, they had agreed to this first meeting that was proposed to all parents whose children entered treatment. During this meeting, Paolo, who at the age of six months expressed all his vitality and desire to know the world, was sitting happily on his dad's lap. He had a nice face, a lively one, with round cheeks that brought to mind advertisements for baby products.

After having talked about how the diagnosis that they had received placed them in a difficult situation, in a realm of confidentiality and secrecy that they were struggling to get out of, the parents began to formulate some hypotheses on what to say – how to talk about Paolo to others and even to his sister, who was ten years old. The sister was experiencing what was happening at home since Paolo's birth, trying to adapt to an atmosphere of pain and reserve without making demands.

After a little while, the mother loosened up and – supported by her husband, who seemed less rigid than at first – talked about how she had felt down when, several days after having returned home with her baby from the hospital where he was born, she had been told by phone that she had to take him to another hospital the following day, in order to begin the medical treatment that had also brought her here today. The idea of the baby's illness hung over her like a menacing shadow, even in this situation in which remedies were available and expectations for the quality of his life were comparable to those of a child without pathology.

> I see that my son is a child who grows and develops well, but in some part of me deep inside, there is always doubt that his beautiful cheeks and his vitality may perhaps be excessive and due to the medications that he takes,

she says. The father listens and comforts her, reminding her that their daughter had a similar countenance when she was Paolo's age and of how happy that made them.

"The illness ruined everything," the mother said, adding, "I know it isn't rational, but I can't stop this internal rumination; we hope that will become possible over time."

While Paolo played calmly, apparently indifferent to what was happening around him, my impression was that there was a slight loosening of the dark and encapsulated pain, which seemed to be poised over the family like a grey cloud, casting a wordless sadness over the parents, Paolo, and his sister. Later on, they decided on their own that by now it was time for the sister to know her little brother had a gland that didn't produce a certain substance and that because of this, he would have to be treated with a medication; every four months he would have lab tests to determine the necessary dosage.

It is this that we must take care of – the cloud that, like a filter, impedes Paolo's mother from seeing his healthy and lively part, which is typically expressed in behaviours precisely at his age. His physical problems can be coped with, but if the pain afflicting his mother is not recognized and considered, then that pain – how can it be treated?

The appearance of a physical illness often represents the resurgence of a traumatic condition that the ill child himself sometimes risks personifying, leading the parent to react to it with all the mechanisms that are really a reaction to the trauma, the negation, the repression, the split. This last leads to the coexistence of mental states that are difficult to reconcile with one another.

Shirley Hoxter (1986) speaks of a "black cloud" that characterizes the experience of some patients and that consists of states of "knowing and not knowing" that interfere with a full integration of feelings and thoughts about one's own condition, which could lead to an overpowering of the ego's capacity to cope. According to this author, these states of "knowing and not knowing," which can coexist side by side but cannot be integrated, can create a great deal of confusion for those who must treat them. For many children, the "black cloud," the traumatic dimension, is experienced as the repetition of a recent trauma, according to the different times of the trauma (described in a separate chapter).

Hoxter maintains that it is quite disconcerting to discover that a communication's content at a given moment conveys security, and, a moment afterward, the same content can represent a threat to the patient. The traumatic dimension suddenly emerges without advance notice, often causing intense fears to arise and, at times, resulting in a flight from contact. According to Hoxter, it is important that clinicians not collude with the denial of illness, but it is equally important that the new encounter experienced as traumatic is not forcibly pushed to occur, analogous to plunging a scalpel into a patient. "Sensitive modulation may be required to enable the repetitions of trauma to lead towards integration rather than to further repetitions of splitting and repression – or overwhelming despair" (Hoxter 1986, p. 95).

Balint (1969) developed this concept, describing trauma as structured in three phases. In the first phase, the immature child is dependent on the adult and, even though frustrations can occur that can lead to irritation and sometimes to rage, the relationship between the child and the adult is essentially one of faith.

In the second phase, the adult, contrary to the child's expectations, does something highly exciting, frightening, or painful; this can happen one time, suddenly, or in a repetitive way and can also relate to an event, an illness, or an incident that happens within the relationship.

Conclusion of the trauma happens in the third phase, when the child approaches the adult with the desire to locate the meaning of what has happened and a continuity of the relationship and now tries to obtain a measure of understanding, recognition, and comfort. That often happens because, in turn pained or traumatized or to avoid new suffering for the child, the adult behaves as though nothing has happened.

If the adult does not take in and confirm the perceptions that the child experiences, the latter lives an experience of confusion that can lead him to enclose himself within a private area of dissociation defined by borders that are made up of the questions that one takes for granted as having no answer or that can hide irreparable reality.

Balint's outline, which seems to me exemplary for its clarity, actually appears to be a systematization of concepts that owe their origins to the ideas of Ferenczi, to whom Balint refers.

Ferenczi believed that trauma, more than from quantitatively daunting elements, stems from the adult's failure to support the child's search for meaning. The adult's denial, silence, and negation about the child's experience give rise to split areas, not integrated into affective experiences or into thought processes.

> Should the quality and quantity of suffering exceed the person's powers of comprehension, then one capitulates; one endures no longer; it is no longer worthwhile to combine these painful things into a unit, and one is split into pieces. I do not suffer any more, indeed I cease to exist, at least as a complete ego. The individual component parts can suffer each by itself.
>
> [Ferenczi 1932, p. 170]

This concept is taken up again by Bokanowski, who maintains that:

> Disqualification by the object (the child's mother or some other close figure) is tantamount to mental rape, leading to paralysis of the ego or to the slow death of mental life. . . . "Trauma," then, is the result of a lack of appropriate response by the object in a situation of distress; as a result, the child's ego is mutilated for all time. This creates a permanently traumatic state and a feeling of helplessness (*Hilflosigkeit*), which may be reactivated at any future point in the individual's life at the slightest provocation.
>
> [Bokanowski 2005, p. 254]

When the experience assumes the emotional flavour of a trauma, it involves the consolidation of massive defensive systems, with important repercussions that also pertain to defining the sense of identity with a limitation, an inhibition, or a distortion of aspects of the ego and an alteration of the sense of self.

Gianna Polacco Williams (1997) reflects on the "double deprivation" relative to children who, beyond being subjected to external deprivations, experience further deprivation from the moment that these conditions lead them to an identification with a depriving internal object and to an operationalization of defensive self-destructive manoeuvres. In the case of a physical illness, this concept seems to hold its validity intact: the child, beyond not being helped to give meaning to what is happening to him and to his body, identifies with the parent's attitude toward his illness, taking on as his own the attitude of nonsincerity and the lack of authentic communication.

Rosenfeld (1978), too, referring to the borderline experience, identifies some traumatic experiences that underlie these patients' experiences. Referring to that work, De Masi also summarizes Rosenfeld's position:

> It is his conviction that prolonged suffering, such as what occurs when a small child feels that he might die (from somatic illness that involves acute physical suffering, as well) and doesn't receive an empathic response on the part of the environment, forms an early nucleus of potential self-destructivity.
>
> [De Masi 2002, p. 51, translation by G. Atkinson]

While in clinical interviews, adolescents tend to minimize their conditions in relation to how their parents see them; in situations in which the pathology entails areas of secrecy and reserve, the situation is turned upside down, and with a sort of pitiful blindness, the parents tend to have a representation of their children that is much less problematic than what they actually experience.

The parents seem to live inside a delusional conviction of having successfully kept their sons or daughters outside of a painful reality.

According to the mother, a sensitive person and apparently emotionally close to her daughter, Jennifer, age 15, knew everything about her clinical conditions – about infertility and the fact of not having either a uterus or ovaries – except what pertained to the Y chromosome, since they planned to inform her about this when she was a little older.

As parents, they had experienced as very difficult the period in which they had discovered the androgen insensitivity syndrome,[1] following Jennifer's recovery from a suspected inguinal hernia. The treating surgeon, in examining the patient, had turned to the mother and exclaimed: "But madam, this child is a boy." Little by little, the parents had overcome the situation and now felt calmer, partly because they viewed their daughter as reasonably calm. Jennifer had many friends, good scholastic performance, and a good social life; they thought that she was coping very well with the additional needs that her condition imposed on her.

The patient had come for an endocrine check-up every six months ever since her condition had been diagnosed at two months of age. In the course of her third year, she had had gonads removed, and at six, a neo-vagina had been constructed for her. At puberty she had embarked on hormonal therapy.

The Meeting with Jennifer

While I had a conversation with the mother, which I came out of with the feeling of facing a situation in which there was attentive and sincere parental involvement – very different from the reserved manner that characterizes the interventions of many other parents – a colleague had a meeting with Jennifer.

The patient presented as a charming, attractive girl, tall and with exquisitely feminine features.

Although Jennifer was at first hesitant toward her, the psychologist said that she had ended up speaking almost without interruption for an hour and a half, alternating between giving intimate accounts, emotional revelations, and outbursts of tears. She appeared to be sensitive and alert, an adolescent who was coping with the awareness of her pathology with the great regret of one who has no one with whom to talk about it. She struggled to speak about it to her mother; for Jennifer, the best person to talk to would have been someone older who had experienced the same problem.

When she was asked why she had come to the hospital, Jennifer tended to be vague, to close herself up – appearing a little embarrassed – and to not want to face the discussion. One sentence, however, had been enough to make her burst into desperate tears, and she had begun to relate that she "will never have menstrual periods and can never have babies." Yes, she had been told that she could adopt children, "but they will never really be mine." As noted, she had come to the hospital regularly every six months, ever since she was little, but only for about two years had her mother explained to her the reason for the visits and the necessity of her pills. She was aware that, if this had been said to her earlier, she might not have understood things because she had been too little. When she had asked her mother, one day in the car her mother had spoken to her about it, and she had tried to make her see "all the pros and cons of this thing." Jennifer had started to cry at once, but she had not immediately understood what her mother meant by "the practical consequences." She needed some time to understand, allowing it to be inferred that she had not foreseen the suffering that the awareness would bring her and perhaps she had not yet understood all that her condition implied.

At home, Jennifer didn't speak to anyone. Not with her brother because she feared that, since the two had friends in common, he might let something slip out to a friend – or with her father, who was up-to-date on the situation but with whom she had not had an occasion to bring up the matter. Her mother – even though she had not forbidden it – always told her not to say anything to anyone except persons whom she could absolutely trust, because someone could use "this thing" to cause her harm.

Every now and then, her mother tried to initiate a conversation, especially when they went to the hospital, one of the few times when they managed to be alone, but Jennifer tried to avoid it. She didn't want to talk about her situation because then she felt worse, even though her thoughts often revolved around it, and an intense need to share these thoughts with someone emerged in an overarching way. Her mother tried as much as she could not to reveal to Jennifer her own suffering in regard to this problem, but Jennifer had understood that, for all her mother's efforts, she did suffer. At any rate, according to her, the mother didn't know how much Jennifer herself suffered from her problem because she hid this from her.

At school, Jennifer was uncomfortable when her friends talked about menstruation and she felt different, even though she told her companions that she had had her periods for some time. Once it happened that during a lesson, there was a discussion about having children, and she had started to cry; since then she had always tried to avoid the topic. The tears flowed again when she told about these things. She said that she always tried not to think about it, but even when she simply saw a child, she "felt uneasy." In the session, she burst out crying again, thinking that she would never be able to have "my own. Yes, I will be able to adopt, and it's beautiful to adopt children, but I'll never be able to have them."

Jennifer did not have a best friend or a friend whom she could confide in, partly because she feared that, living in a town in which everyone knew each other, everyone would come to know about her problem.

She told of having undergone three surgeries: one at two months of age, one at two years, and a third at six years. She didn't remember anyone or anything about these interventions. She knew that she had had them to remove an inguinal hernia, and during one of these, the doctors had noticed that she did not have ovaries.

Jennifer intuited, however, that the truth was something else, that there was much more, but for now she didn't yet feel like asking for further explanations. She said, "Maybe I'll ask when I'm eighteen and will be better able to understand, and I'll have studied what an inguinal hernia actually is."

She had an enormous fear of what doctors would be able to tell her regarding the interventions that she had undergone, as though now she couldn't tolerate another truth that would upset her as she had been upset when her mother had spoken with her about it. She maintained that she still had time, that she should wait another few years in order to better experience what she already knew before she faced up to additional painful information. The doctor who had followed her when she was little had told her that when she wanted to and when she felt ready, she could call him and speak with him about it. Every now and then she would have a wish to do this, but she thought it was still too early. She was afraid to ask because she didn't know "how these things might be said to me, because the way in which things are said is also important – but especially because I don't know what they might tell me."

Jennifer had two scars, one on her hip and one in her groin area that bothered her a great deal. At the beach, people would ask her questions that always made her think about her problem, even though she replied that she had had a cyst and a hernia removed, and then she would try to change the subject. But the scars always made her think about her problem.

When their meeting ended, Jennifer hugged and kissed the psychologist, smiling at her.

I thought about recounting the process of these two meetings, which had required a little more than three hours of work, because they seem to me to encapsulate, at least in condensed form, many of the emotional problems linked to conditions in which variations in sexual development are present.

After that meeting, however, there was still much work to be done; some years passed, and there had still not been a chance to open up a small passage into this dimension of intense suffering. The mother continued to carry the cross that she bore, and her daughter did the same, both dwelling in an area of great loneliness.

Unfortunately, we were forced to note that, in cases like this one, if the truth is not told on the right occasion, when the emotional dimension feels warm, it is then difficult to identify the optimal moment in the future. It is more probable that a cloud of collusion will replace a relationship based on authenticity.

Sandra Filippini (2005), in her book on perverse relationships, highlighted a key moment beyond which the relationship assumes pathological characteristics, passing a point of no return. I believe that that moment, the time of the first infraction, consists of the first omission of truth and that the hope of tomorrow bringing a more favourable moment may be only the first step in a chain of omissions and pain.

A pain can be so great as to be unrecognizable in its existence, and therefore it is denied.

At eight years of age, Luisa was brought to the hospital because she was beginning to develop and mature, and after a series of exams, she was diagnosed with a form of congenital adrenal hyperplasia.[2] She is now 20, a university student, and this is the first time she has been offered the chance to talk about what she experienced during the past 12 years.

Luisa is deeply disappointed by how her case has been managed. She believes that her attitude of mistrusting others, especially her parents and doctors, has for years contributed to her rejection of her condition and her desire not to know too much about it.

In order not to cause her suffering, Luisa's parents did not tell her in detail about what her condition truly was. Luisa said:

> I still don't know very well what my situation is. I grew up with the idea that it was something temporary – that I had to take pills for a while, for something that sooner or later would pass. Then, over the years, I became more aware that there was something that wasn't going well, and in the face of my parents' silence, I tried to learn about it on my own; I was by then a big girl. I was so disappointed that I reacted by refusing to learn any more about it. Little by little, I'm beginning to accept all that it means, but it is very difficult; there are a ton of problems – like when I'm with friends on vacation and have to pay attention to the timing of my medications and where my purse is, because if by chance my friends see my pills inside, I won't know how to explain. All this not talking has meant that I've accepted things at a later point, and my growth has been influenced by my parents who don't talk about it and by doctors whose talk is too difficult to follow. Now I would like to be informed by a doctor who is aware that he's speaking with someone who didn't go to medical school. I've been glad to talk to you about these things, but this meeting should have happened twelve years ago.

It is also true that it's never too late; there is always time to bridge silences and interrupted dialogues, as we can see from a letter I received from a mother who only over time found an alternative way for her and her daughter to cope with the daughter's problem.

Dear Doctor,

I am the person who came to you several months ago to speak with you about my daughter, who has androgen insensitivity syndrome. I write to thank you. Our meeting allowed me to begin a small revolution in my mind and in my heart.

For months, I carried around informational brochures that you had given me wherever we went, even on vacation, though I managed to read only a few pages at a time, as though I needed a long time and great care in coming to grips with the emotions of my story that had been silenced for too long.

I often found myself thinking of your calm yet active tone of voice, and your light and delicate smile, when you explained to me the importance of not keeping certain secrets.

It was the first time in almost nineteen years that I felt (not only knew) that there could be another way of taking care of my daughter Lidia and of her development and growth, a way that would give both her and me the possibility of clearer and deeper exchanges with each other. I could think about telling her – and also telling myself – the details of her (and our) story, without the subtle censuring brought on by fear, by shame and pain.

A few weeks ago, I finally explained to Lidia the things that she still didn't know about her situation (especially the matter of the XY chromosomal structure).

She had intuited these things, but in such a confused and messed-up way that my account was for her a relief, and a good occasion for us to feel close to one another.

As for me, I feel I've been suddenly liberated from a trap that had me bound and gagged, and very frightened, for too many years. And my wounds have become like small openings – new "windows" from which to observe the world and also my young girl, who is now becoming a woman.

I think that your way of welcoming me and speaking with me has greatly contributed to making me take these important steps recently, as though you had taken me by the hand and helped me find the path out of a dark and silent forest in which I'd been rather lost.

And so, thank you from the heart!

The Doctor's Pain

It is not easy to communicate a complex diagnosis, for many reasons – first, because every specialist is an expert in his own particular field, and in facing these situations he often relies on his own goodwill, experience, and personal sensitivity, without being able to trust in shared methods or a plan that has been arranged with colleagues.

An early way to be helped is not to work alone but to be able to count on a group of colleagues with whom to share not only the clinical content but emotional problems as well.

The most innovative experiences in this area have highlighted how the communication of the diagnosis might be closely tied to the relational dimension between doctor and patient. And when one speaks of a relational dimension, one leaves behind a unilaterally directed action that runs exclusively from the caregiver to the patient. Instead, it means taking account of the fact that sometimes communicating a diagnosis is an emotionally burdensome experience for the one who must accomplish it as well; although they are experts, even doctors, psychologists, and nurses are not immune to the contagion of intense emotions with which they come into contact.

We often look for tools that may facilitate communication, and psychoanalysis has something to tell us about these tools, because with the primary one – communication – the fact that we are the ones who must communicate the presence of pathology is somewhat reflective of a failure of the mechanisms that have led us to choose a health care profession.

We frequently notice that we have been led to make our professional choices based on deep motivations that have to do with the desire to take care of aspects of ourselves that have been wounded, sickened, unpleasant, or possibly neglected.

An author whom we have already encountered in previous chapters, Isabel Menzies Lyth (1960), emphasized that in the situations we face in clinical practice, there is an impressive similarity to situations of fantasy life present in every individual at very deep and primitive mental levels. She maintains that one of the most important motivations in this professional choice may be the desire to develop subliminatory activities of curing the sick and, through these, to better master anxiety-provoking childhood situations, modifying pathological anxiety and arriving at professional maturity.

In the initial motivations for many professions, which then the experience mitigates and makes more realistic, there is a desire to also take care of ourselves as we take care of others, restoring a state of health and well-being.

When we must communicate a diagnosis, this fantasy breaks up and forces us to come to terms with the unconscious emotional components that we carry inside.

Considerable work is required to stay in contact with feelings that it would be easy to discharge, almost to evacuate, entrusting them to the patient and, once our work is done, distancing ourselves from them. Much work is required in order to transform these irrational components, remaining in contact, creating a connection with the person that continues over time and will convey the feeling of being able to cope with the situation together. This means trying to recognize, accepting, and containing the mental pain of persons with whom professionals come into contact through meetings that aim to offer them a mental space where their anxieties and their feelings can eventually be named, communicated, and shared.

That is not always easy because, as Hoxter (1986) reminds us, "those who are themselves traumatised can offer the child neither protection from the re-emergence of fright nor developmental experiences enabling the integration of trauma". And in fact:

> Child psychotherapists are not immune from such defensive reactions to the traumatised child. Yet we cannot work with traumatised patients unless we can analyse and integrate our own experiences of trauma, so that we ourselves are not more than momentarily traumatised by the impact of our patients' trauma.
>
> (p. 91)

A way to protect ourselves from trauma is to assume particularly active attitudes, yet it is important to respect the timing and sensibility of individual persons and not to put ourselves forward to be perceived as omniscient experts – something that would end up merely reinforcing the experience of inadequacy in the people whom we would like to help.

To summarize, years of experience in communicating diagnoses – and especially in "giving bad news" – have revealed two factors of basic importance, closely related to each other. The first is that, as we have seen, especially in the past, there was a tendency not to tell everything but to keep the person in the dark about his condition. Underlying some of the omissions was the assumption of being able to know what was good and what was not good for the person; i.e., "for his own good, it is better that he not know." Over time this attitude was seen to represent an actual extortion of the person's right to know and to be responsible for his own destiny, a violation of an inalienable individual right and of a first attempt to take charge of his own condition.

The second factor relates to not taking into account the emotional impact of the communication to be given on the person who must communicate the diagnosis. Although this person is thinking about saving the patient from what he imagines to be emotional suffering from possible trauma, in reality, he is saving himself from it, often adopting an evacuative style that amounts to liberating himself from his own burden of anxiety. Unfortunately, he ends up handing down that anxiety precisely to the person whose suffering he had wanted to avoid.

To overcome these difficulties, especially in more complex cases – but every case is complex for the person involved and requires special attention, even apparently more simple ones – the necessity of group work must be avowed, work that, as much as possible, meets the patient's needs globally. The central point seems to be collaboration among the various professionals who work with patients, on the model of the "Clinical Conference" that geneticists propose for genetic consultations (Leuzinger-Bohleber et al. 2008; Astori et al. 2016), in which the individual case and the counselling relationship between doctor and patient are discussed among clinicians, often including psychologists and psychoanalysts.

One must aim for a consulting style that encourages the professional's capacity to use understandable language, to be in contact with unconscious feelings and the fantasies of those in treatment with him, permitting the doctor-patient couple to work through their emotional situation and mentally contain the feelings that arise from stressful circumstances, in order to avoid reactions that can lead to acting out.

The meetings must have a dedicated place and time; they must not have a paternalistic flavour or a directive slant – which must not be confused with a forum in which suggestions may be given. Here the clinician gives information and, step by step, tries to explore and allow the patient's abilities and skills to emerge, such that he can come to his own decision.

This availability to listen more than to talk represents a technique requiring skills and the presence of a relevant, established group. It presupposes that those who do this work will have developed not only competence in medical and genetic techniques but will also possess sufficient skills to be capable of maintaining contact with the human and interpersonal problems that arise in the communication of biomedical data.

The various steps along the journey of communication assume, first of all, an acceptance and an attentive listening to the patient on the part of the person who hopes to be able to remain an established interlocutor who accompanies people through the course of understanding and acceptance of the diagnosis and who, over time, makes themselves available for further encounters and clarifications.

Another relevant point is the presence of a multiprofessional group to whom the clinician can present the case and with whom he can question himself about clinical aspects and the emotional and psychological implications. The mind of the group – the group's psychic apparatus (Kaës 1999) – makes it capable of supporting the clinician who is charged with the situation and modality of communication. In other words, the group confirms the clinician's medical competence and helps him stay in contact with the patient's pain.

Even though it can be taken for granted that, for reasons that we have in part seen earlier, a correct way of communicating the diagnosis does not exist – that at best, this represents a goal toward which to strive, an objective that we can approach to a greater or lesser degree – the way of communicating the diagnosis becomes a fundamentally important factor for subsequent necessary treatments as well.

First and foremost, it is important to emphasize once again that the communication of a diagnosis cannot be approached only in rational terms. Rather, it is a process that requires time before a person or a couple might be capable of facing the relevant choices with at least minimal rationality.

In the case of children, powerful psychological defensive processes in the parents filter the data. They may deny it or distort it and require time before becoming even partially aware of what they have been told.

It is undoubtedly a burdensome task for the doctor, one that requires competence, sensitivity, experience, a sense of one's own limits and a group of established colleagues with whom to share the choices to be made. This is true also because, in those moments, the parents frequently attribute to the doctor the status of a god – omnipotence – and the capacity to anticipate developments that are almost impossible to predict. They may even almost credit him with having the possibility of arranging life or death, at times asking him for the definitive word.

This responsibility of a doctor's goes beyond his capabilities and is not easy to accept – a responsibility that is not new and that has to do with the compulsion for knowledge inherent in human nature, expressed through myths since the origin of humanity. For example, the ancient Greek poet Hesiod, in his didactic poem "The Works and Days" (written about 700 BC), speaking of illnesses, told us that these come to men spontaneously by day and by night – "bringing misfortunes to mortal beings" silently, because the wise Zeus "took the word away from them." But myths also tell us of man's need to know. Similarly, when man lived in a primitive state, free of needs and of illness, Prometheus stole sparks from the gods – the fire of knowledge – and handed it down to men.

Zeus, irritated with Prometheus, wanted to take revenge on humankind as well, because of its ambition to know more than the human condition permitted, entering into fields of knowledge that until then were the exclusive domain of the gods. Zeus asked Hephaestus to use water and earth to construct for him the body of a young girl, Pandora, called by this name because all the gods had given her a gift. Laden with gifts and flattery, she was sent as a present to man, who gladly accepted her, but when she opened the box that she carried with her, all the world's illnesses and troubles flew out. Hurrying to close the lid of the box, Pandora managed to keep inside only hope, which she allowed to come out later; thus the world, destroyed by misfortunes, could then come back to life.

As we see at a distance of more than 2,500 years, the questions posed by mankind at the time of the ancient Greek myths are still, in certain ways, those of today.

The information that we have at our disposal today thanks to technological tools allows us to explore areas that were previously the realm of the gods. Today we can push ourselves to the deepest abyss of genomes and know an individual's most intimate genetic determinants.

The power of the technical tools that we make use of is not accompanied by an adjustment of the instruments needed to evaluate the mode of communication with those involved or to evaluate the consequences of acts that are not always fully esteemed.

Pushed by the need to deepen our knowledge even more, we must try to refine our tools of communication as well, in order to avoid – in contrast to Pandora – being dazzled by our technical capabilities and, somewhat slow in closing the lid of the box that we have opened, risking the disappearance even of hope in the persons whom we would like to help.

Notes

1   Androgen insensitivity syndrome (AIS) is a condition that relates to the development of the genital and reproductive system. See the chapter on variations of sexual differentiation.
2   Congenital adrenal hyperplasia (CAH) is an endocrine disorder arising from a genetic deficit that impairs the production of one or more adrenal hormones. The disorder must be attentively monitored, and the missing hormones must be synthetically integrated with multiple daily doses. See also the chapter on variations in sexual differentiation.

References

Astori, S., Ferruta, A. & Mariotti, C. (2016). *La diagnosi genetica: un dialogo per la cura. Storie cliniche negli Alberi della vita [The Genetic Diagnosis: A Dialogue for the Cure. Clinical Stories in the "Alberi della Vita"]*. Milano: Franco Angeli.

Balint, M. (1969). Trauma and object relationship. *Int. J. Psychoanal.*, 50:429–435.

Bokanowski, T. (2005). Variations on the concept of traumatism: Traumatism, traumatic, trauma. *Int. J. Psychoanal.*, 86:251–265.

De Masi, F. (2002). *Il limite dell'esistenza: un contributo psicoanalitico al problema della caducità della vita [The Limit of Existence: A Psychoanalytic Contribution to the Problem of the Decline of Life]*. Torino: Bollati Boringhieri.

Ferenczi, S. (1932). *The Clinical Diary of Sándor Ferenczi*, ed. J. Dupont, trans. M. Balint & N. Z. Jackson. Cambridge, MA/London: Harvard University Press, 1985.

Ferro, A. (2002). *Seeds of Illness, Seeds of Recovery*, trans. P. Slotkin. Hove, UK: Brunner-Routledge, 2005.

Filippini, S. (2005). *Relazioni perverse. La violenza psicologica nella coppia [Perverse Relationships: Psychological Violence in the Couple]*. Milano: Franco Angeli.

Freud, S. (1915). Mourning and melancholia. *S. E.*, 14.

Harris, M. & Meltzer, D. (2013). *The Educational Role of the Family: A Psychoanalytical Model*. ISD LLC.

Hoxter, S. (1986). Significance of trauma in the difficulties encountered by physically disabled children. *J. Child Psychother.*, 12:87–102.

Joffe, W. G. & Sandler, J. (1965). Notes on pain, depression and individualization. *Psychoanal. Study Child*, 20:394–424.

Kaës, R. (1999). *Les Théories Psychianalitique du Group*. Paris: Press Universitaires de France.

Kaës, R. (2012). *Le teorie psicoanalitiche del Gruppo*. Roma: Borla.

Leuzinger-Bohleber, M., Engels, E.-M. & Tsiantos, J., eds. (2008). *The Janus Face of Prenatal Diagnosis*. London: Karnac.

Menzies Lyth, I. (1960). A case-study in the functioning of social systems as a defence against anxiety. *Hum. Relat.*, 13(2):95–121.

Polacco Williams, G. (1997). *Internal Landscapes and Foreign Bodies: Eating Disorders and Other Pathologies*. New York: Routledge.

Rosenfeld, H. (1978). Notes on the psychopathology and psychoanalytic treatment of some borderline patients. *Int. J. Psychoanal.*, 58:215–239.

Chapter 5

Child Psychoanalysis

Giorgia, at the age of four years and three months, did not want to be called by her name; she said that she was an animal, a dog or a fox, and she wanted to be treated accordingly.

She expressed herself in this way especially with persons whom she didn't know or didn't know very well. A few days earlier, she had asserted to some family friends that she was a cheetah, had pretended to unsheathe her claws, and said that if people continued to bother her, she would kill everyone.

Giorgia's mother had reached the point of feeling ashamed to take her out due to her frequent conflictual crises and her need to always be the centre of attention, which reminded the mother of the "worst" aspect of her husband's character. In these real, "head-to-head" encounters, the mother had the feeling that the child did it precisely to be unpleasant, as though she were searching in every way possible to attract her mother's attention and intervention.

At our first meeting, the mother also related that, at around 18 months of age, Giorgia had suddenly stopped eating for almost a month, at the same time that she started preschool and after the birth of a little cousin of whom she seemed to be jealous. Her condition of intense asthenia had raised the possibility of some physical illness and had required a hospital stay. After a lengthy admission, Giorgia had eaten very little for almost six months and then, little by little, she had resumed eating. Her mother's account continued with a description of a child who wasn't easy, who always tended to oppose her and who didn't want to urinate when she was told to; at times she did it on the ground like an animal, and even punishments and severe scolding were not successful in dissuading her from her intentions.

When Giorgia was brought to preschool, she cried, and when her schoolmates called her by name, she got angry, continuing to insist that she was a fox. Her mother, though being very worried and involved in her daughter's difficulties, seemed to be far from any real understanding of them. One could hear desperation in her voice – a sense of shame and impotence around her relationship with her daughter that she could not allow herself to express.

The parents lived in two different cities: the mother in Bologna, where she worked in an office, while the father lived in another region, where he was

DOI: 10.4324/9781003252238-6

responsible for a building site. The mother found the family arrangement unsatisfactory, but she expressed no clear intent to interrupt or change it.

The parental couple presented as an abstract entity, apparently not built around a solid relationship. Before their marriage they had gotten along well, but with Giorgia's birth, their rapport had deteriorated; according to the mother, they had "counted their chickens before they were hatched." The father, whom I met with only one time – ostensibly because of logistical difficulties but in reality because of his marginal role in the family constellation – did not seem able to see his daughter's problems. According to the mother, he was never comfortable in his role as a dad, and he had gradually become more detached from the management of their family life. The child, whom the father had begun to know when she was five months old, now saw him on weekends, and on those occasions they were frequently in conflict.

For the mother, Giorgia had been a calm baby during the first year of life; she slept well and ate adequately. She was breastfed until the sixth month, when the mother had returned to work and Giorgia had remained at home, usually with her grandmother.

The mother believed she had done enough for her daughter, being with her whenever she could and taking her to the grandmother's, but now she found herself recognizing that Giorgia had been "tossed around like a package." At about 18 months of age, she had been enrolled in preschool, after the summer in which the cousin whom she had always been jealous of was born. During that period, she had most likely lost some of the care and attention given to her by her grandmother, whose presence had been an important reference point for her.

The problems had manifested in that period, when Giorgia "didn't socialize much," and the presence of some people provoked loud outbursts of crying; it was also the time when her refusal of food began, along with her first hospitalization.

In our initial observational meetings, Giorgia presented as a little woman, both in her clothing and her behaviour. Her nail polish, more than child's play, seemed an attempt to appear older, as did her "grown-up" discussions – in which, if one asked the reason for some of the words she used, an unclear distinction between fantasy and reality emerged, as well as contents typical of a younger child. Her drawings, too, were childish for her age, and when Giorgia did not have full control of the situation, she seemed gripped by deep anxiety. Not being able to express her emotions directly, she tried to conform to an image of an older child, with a forward thrust that left behind her more childish aspects – a high cost for keeping her defensive organization in efficient working order.

When these childish traits emerged, Giorgia muddied the waters in a strategy similar to the one her mother used: she talked at length in superficial discussions that seemed to have the aim only of distancing herself from the emotions that upset her. At other times, very regressed behaviours emerged that scared her, such as when she had the feeling of being little without being able to keep her more primitive aspects in check.

Giorgia's exhibitionistic behaviours, which could have been characteristic of a child some years older than she, had an intensity such that they made one think of an attempt to hide an image of a little self, unappreciated and neglected, both from herself and from others. Her aggressive behaviours, too – at times decisively provocative – expressed the discomfort of a child who was desperately trying to keep control of a situation, not believing that the relationship with her mother was reliable, or attracting her attention even if it led to punishment.

In this situation, everything led up to a view of the child's weak internal representation of herself, something that brought to mind Winnicott's (1965) *false self*. Likewise, there was a similarly unstable investment of internal objects, including the representation of the mother. Her presence inside the child was not taken for granted but was continually exposed to an ongoing worry about having to keep the connection with her alive.

It was not easy to organize Giorgia's difficulties into a precise nosographic picture due to the psychic plasticity of her age group and the variability of her symptoms. "Neurotic" terminology, referring to the presence of psychic conflicts in individuals with a sufficiently cohesive personality structure, was not terribly useful, nor was "psychotic" appropriate, alluding to persons for whom the relationship between internal and external reality appeared precarious. I preferred to focus on the more flexible concept of *developmental disharmony*, which, drawing on the language of Misès and Quemada (2002), consists of a personality disturbance whose seriousness and whose possible obstacles to subsequent development go beyond the limit of neuroses but without there being a rupture in reality testing that could lead into the area of the psychoses.

After four meetings with Giorgia, in a new meeting of *restoration* – a term with which, in psychological jargon, one defines the act of "restoring" or "giving back" to the parents what it had been possible to understand in meetings with their child – I communicated to the mother that, in my opinion, there were reasons to propose psychotherapeutic treatment for Giorgia. It also seemed important to more deeply explore with the mother herself some aspects of their relationship.

Actually, even though the mother had been very involved and made tremendous efforts, she did not seem aware of her own pain and desperation that underlay a generic discomfort in her relationship with her daughter. For the mother, Giorgia's birth seems to have reactivated unresolved difficulties that brought her back to her own childhood and the relationship with her parents. In other words, it appeared necessary to dig deeper in understanding the relationship between the mother and her family of origin, in order to see to what degree it might be possible for this woman to have a relationship with her daughter that wasn't unduly influenced by the history of her connections to her own mother and siblings.

Once I had ascertained that my proposal of psychotherapy would be favourably received, it was clear that it would not be possible for me to see the child and her mother simultaneously, and so I referred the mother to a colleague with whom she could begin treatment that, over time, might develop into real psychotherapy. In the meantime, I had begun to see Giorgia once a week, within my position at the hospital. In the beginning, all her play activities were aimed at keeping the situation under control. When I spoke to her, she seemed to emotionally acknowledge what I wanted to communicate, even though she also seemed not to care and would continue her own discourse, undaunted, sometimes speaking over me.

Over the course of some months, Giorgia's most obvious symptoms were somewhat reduced; she went to preschool more willingly, and the teachers noticed improvement in her relationships with peers. In her drawings, I noted an increase in her ability to give graphic form to her thoughts, even though she often tended to immediately erase or destroy what she had drawn.

Giorgia's mother was also helped by her therapy. She got better at seeing her daughter's behaviours as expressions of a younger child's neediness, and she no longer competed with her, as she had done before in an attitude similar to one she might have shown toward an adult whom she was standing up to.

In therapy, Giorgia often demonstrated keen interest in a multicolored jar on my desk, despite having an identical one at her own disposal. With these frequently transgressive and provocative behaviours, she seemed to me to be grasping some of the thoughts that troubled her about our relationship – for example, about the children who might later take her place in my office; evidently, for her, the colours of the jar were a manifestation of these children's presence. My attempts to talk about her moods relative to these themes seemed not to obtain any confirmation, apparently.

For personal reasons, on one occasion I had to cancel a session. At the next session, Giorgia looked for any excuse whatsoever not to come into my office; the last was that her mother, who had accompanied her, had hurt herself while getting out of the car. Once Giorgia was finally in the room, she overturned the box containing her toys with a loud crash, and then began to talk about which animals could or could not be nearby.

When I tried to say something to her, she said that she wanted to leave the room to go to the bathroom. I told her that she could leave if she wanted to, of course, but she might do better if we found a way to confront what she was feeling that seemed to be upsetting her. When she answered that she didn't feel well, almost in a kidding way, I suggested that she lie down on the little couch. She did this and, once lying down, she relaxed and put a finger in her mouth like a much younger child.

Giorgia lay down for some time. It was the first time that I had not seen her moving about actively. For a while she remained silent, allowing a little bit of saliva to drip from her lips, something that reminded her of a game she had played when she was smaller – trying to control the quantity of saliva that she let out of one side of her mouth without it falling. Her need to go to the bathroom had passed, she no longer wanted to go outside, and the session ended calmly.

After this session, two more with a very similar process followed, even though the moments of agitation were more intense. In one session, Giorgia talked to me about eating and about the fact that she had been good; she had eaten everything. We were approaching a vacation period, and her mother had requested an appointment in which she took the opportunity to congratulate me because she had learned from a mutual acquaintance that there was a new baby in my family (the reason for my absence a few sessions earlier). Immediately afterward, the mother recounted that, for about 20 days, Giorgia had refused to eat, and only during the prior several days had she ingested anything. This period coincided with changes in our sessions, Giorgia's oppositional behaviour, and her temporary refusal to enter my office.

Suddenly, I realized that I was behaving like the mother who failed to see that the reasons for Giorgia's changed mood were all to be found in our relationship. I asked the mother if by chance Giorgia had been updated on the events in my own family, and the mother did not exclude from possibility that she may have spoken of these things in her daughter's presence.

Without warning, a connection had been born between Giorgia's fantasies about other children taking her place, the earlier refusal of food when she was placed in preschool, and the birth of the little cousin who stole from her the cherished time spent with her grandmother. Seeing this connection made the difficulties of our more problematic sessions understandable.

Giorgia had not been able to talk to me about how upset she was by my absence related to a new birth, which reawakened her feelings of exclusion and her fear of again experiencing the suffering she had already been through. It was as though our relationship was "engulfed" by these unexpressed feelings, and so it wasn't easy for her to enter the room and regress to a much younger child who sucked her thumb or who rushed everything, keeping control of the situation in order to protect herself from the emergence of intolerable pain.

Only with time and with the progression of the therapy were we able to talk about how Giorgia had reexperienced within our relationship the pain that had not been fully embraced when she expressed it in the past. Only now could her chaotic emotions take shape – indigestible and undigested feelings that had permeated her – and she could now express her aggression in a more direct way.

The case of Giorgia, which took place in a health care institution – something that is becoming more and more logistically difficult due to reductions in manpower resources, as well as decreased investment in therapeutic interventions that may have a preventative function, in a structured way, in the consolidation of more serious illnesses – adds something to the close relationship between psychoanalysis and health care institutions that we have examined in previous chapters. I thought that the description of a real case could introduce the theme of child psychoanalysis and highlight its crucial contribution to our knowledge of the child's emotional life and to the treatment of developmental pathologies.

Additionally, it can allow us to see how material is condensed within it that has emerged in the course of the historical development of child psychoanalysis, through its contributions and applications to various aspects of the child's experience and his relationships with his parents or those who care for him. From the field of child psychoanalysis, in addition to the development of therapeutic techniques, important contributions have emerged on early mental states, attachment, genitality and its variations, children's institutions, adoption, hospitalization, the consequences of early separation, etc. For these reasons, it can be useful to re-examine the phases of development and evolution in child psychoanalysis, from its origins to the present day.

The Origins of Child Psychoanalysis

Child psychoanalysis focuses on situations in which the child's internal world appears to be blocked, structured in a rigidly pathological way that doesn't allow him to face with sufficient flexibility the current demands of emotional and social reality and those of subsequent developmental phases. In these cases, psychoanalysis proves a necessary tool in modifying the areas of suffering and obstacles to psychic development that have formed the basis of symptomology. In that way, child analysis is different from other forms of therapeutic intervention whose objective is the elimination of symptomatic behaviours.

In order to clarify this difference, we can cite Anna Freud, who described a child who, in order to protect himself from anxiety deriving from conflict between his instinctual wishes and environmental demands, developed an obsessive symptomatology that caused him to always carry a rucksack and have a hat on his head whenever he went out – something that in its compulsive repetition came to be considered by those around him as a disturbance. In the face of adult insistence, the child quickly learned to rid himself of his "rucksack-and-hat" symptom, and he found it less problematic to always keep a pencil in his pocket. As Anna Freud writes:

> From that time he was regarded as normal. He had adapted his mechanism to suit his environment, or at least he concealed it and did not allow it to conflict with other people's requirements. But this did not mean that there was any change in the inner anxiety situation.
>
> [p. 91]

Child psychoanalysis took its first steps discreetly, soon interweaving its path with the development of psychoanalytic thinking, originally aimed at the adult. Already with Sigmund Freud's early writing on the dream (1900) and in his *Three Essays on the Theory of Sexuality* (1905), the child and his development had become a fundamental element of his entire theoretical system. Far from living in an idyllic dimension, the child was described in the *Three Essays* as a network of drive aspects. As the child grew and developed, one could identify "psychic embankments" of modesty, disgust, and morality, and the instinctual desires incompatible with the ego found their passage toward consciousness blocked. The basic defence impeding transit from the unconscious to the preconscious during an early period was represented by repression; when the solution had not been satisfactory, pathology developed, at that time basically organized as "neuroses."

In the years in which Freud described the various phases of psychosexual development, his interest in childhood was mostly theoretical. He was not as directly
focused on drawing therapeutic procedures from it as he was on finding confirmation of the theories he had formulated on the aetiology of the neuroses and on their
link to childhood sexuality.

Freud's first description of a child psychotherapy appears in his work on Little
Hans (1908), in which he described the treatment of a childhood phobia. Max
Graf – a musicologist and writer in the circle of Freud's pupils who had married a
woman who had been in analysis with him – spoke to Freud about his son, Herbert
(Hans), who at three years and nine months developed a fear of being bitten by a
horse. It was not a direct treatment; Freud saw the child only once and indirectly
followed him through the therapy that he conducted with the boy's father, with
his encouragement. To Freud this did not seem strange; indeed, the fact that the
father and the therapist were the same person formed a linchpin of the treatment,
in his opinion.

In this early application of analysis to a child, Freud affirmed that Hans could
accept the therapy because the father's authority was added to that of the therapist,
who agreed to address the child's fears and to alleviate his anxiety. It was not such a
strange thing in that period, given that there was not as much attention as there is today
to preserving the therapeutic setting – that is, to the overall conditions of the therapist's arrangement that permit therapy to take place, whether environmental, temporal, methodologic, etc. Freud himself had in analysis on two occasions his daughter
Anna, his friend Karl Abraham, and Little Hilda, while Melanie Klein analysed all
three of her own children, who later underwent treatments with her colleagues.

Already in 1925, however, the advisability of this practice does not seem to
have been widely shared, if one recalls that Alix Strachey, who had had a meeting
with Lou Andreas Salomé in Berlin, recounted to her husband that Lou

> had the most antiquated ideas . . . from Freud at the time of "Little Hans."
> When she said that the parents were the only proper people to analyse the
> child, a shiver ran down my spine. It seems to me to be the last stronghold of
> the desire of adults to have power over others.
>
> [Grosskurth 1986, p. 135]

At any rate, those early experiences allowed for interpretation of the behaviour
and play of the child, and Freud deepened his study of the genesis of phobia and
identified early therapeutic interventions. Hans's phobia had arisen via the creation of a phobic object through mechanisms of displacement and projection; that
is, he was afraid of his own hostile desires toward his father and had transformed
this into the fear of being bitten by a horse.

This case helped Freud confirm the existence of child sexuality and to develop
childhood theories on the "excrementitious complex" – on the belief that children
are born from the anus, on the fact that both boys and girls are born equipped with
a penis, and that girls are then deprived of the penis through castration. Especially,

the case allowed him to bring into focus the oedipal complex, with the child's attraction to the parent of the opposite sex and the consequent aggressive and exclusionary fantasies toward the other parent.

Freud's intuitions on the child's psychic world were quickly incorporated into a therapeutic perspective on childhood. Early attempts were geared to an application in the pedagogical area of psychoanalytic knowledge having a prophylactic objective. To give an example, Freud wanted to present the case of Little Hans at a 1908 psychoanalytic congress, but he preferred to entrust the job of the introductory remarks to Ferenczi, on the topic of "psychoanalysis and pedagogy," in which the meeting between the two sciences led to a very optimistic vision of the potential of psychoanalysis. If neurosis derived from the sum of predispositional factors and "life changes," a certain kind of education could increase the influence of life chances and, therefore, by acting on the educational system, one could protect children from trauma and anxiety – and as a result, prevent neurosis.

Freud thus championed "psychoanalytic education," a theory that over time demonstrated its limitations, and various experiments were initiated in which attempts were made to apply it: Bernfeld's, at a preschool set up according to psychoanalytic theories at Vienna Baumgarten and Vera Schmidt's, at a psychoanalytic preschool in Moscow.

In Vienna, Hermine Hug-Hellmuth had begun to treat children with a therapy focused on play and on the necessity of creating an emotional rapport with the child's family. Her experiences incorporated one-hour sessions, primarily in children's homes, in which she played together with the child, using his games and trying to help him express his needs and repressed desires, with the aim of securing his trust and thus creating a positive transference.

Hug-Hellmuth died tragically in 1924, however, killed by the 18-year-old nephew who had been her principal patient – and for whom, besides being a therapist, she had also become an oppressive mother. The nephew, after having left prison, sought compensation for damages from Federn, temporary president of the Vienna Psychoanalytic Center, complaining of having been used by Hug-Hellmuth as an object of laboratory experimentation. Her tragic end highlighted the risk of transferential collusion combined with an under-recognized negative transference.

Seen as an area of psychoanalysis particularly adapted to women clinicians – and, due to its proximity to the educational field, being open to those who were not medical doctors – child psychoanalysis, starting in the 1920s, was developed through the activities of Freud's youngest daughter, Anna (Vienna 1895–London 1982) and Melanie Klein (Vienna 1882–London 1960).

The two women's theories were soon destined to take divergent paths, with a conceptual clash that took shape publicly in their remote confrontation when Anna Freud collected her theories into the 1926 essay, "Four Lectures on Child Analysis," to which Klein responded in 1927 with her "Symposium on Child Analysis."

Anna Freud

Anna Freud believed that in child analysis, one must first take account of the child's situation of dependence on the parents, even before what pertains to the therapeutic alliance; the area involving the id, ego, and superego; and the motivations that bring people to therapy. In her opinion, in cases where the child's disturbances do not represent a problem for him but instead are problematic for his parents, the analysis should be preceded by a preparatory phase in which the therapist, through a series of pleasurable activities, must earn the child's benevolent stance.

In Anna Freud's view, child analysis is different from that of the adult in relation to the transference as well. According to classical theory, there was no therapy in which a transference neurosis did not arise to be called out – one in which all the drive forces underlying the patient's symptom ended up directed toward the analyst, and once they were worked through, the symptomatology was reduced. But according to her view, a transference neurosis is not always evident in child therapies, and not everything that the child brings to therapy leads back to the analyst. Indeed, the latter finds himself having to share the child's hateful and loving impulses toward his primary objects, the parents. So the external world influences childhood neurosis and the analysis much more than in the adult because of the direct influence that the parents have over the child. For these same reasons, it isn't possible to analyze the oedipal complex, another key component of the adult analyses of that period.

If in adult therapy, one tries to liberate the motions of the drive from the negative action of repression, thus rendering them available to the superego's influence, in child therapy, with a superego that has not yet solidified, elimination of the drive's influence risks exposing the patient to the mercy of impulses that he isn't capable of dealing with. In order to avoid this, the therapy therefore has to consist of a joint endeavour by both the therapist and the parents.

The child therapist also differs from the adult therapist with respect to the termination of analysis because the adult patient, with a structured ego and superego that can help him cope with the situation, is capable of being primarily responsible for what he does. In the child, the analysis, besides allowing the patient to express unconscious instinctual contents, must aim at "reducing the demands" of a primitive superego, causing the therapist to assume more benign superego functions that, at the conclusion of the analysis, can be entrusted to the parental arena.

In this regard, Anna Freud described the case of an obsessive six-year-old girl whom she had treated. In the course of their sessions, the little girl became more and more lively; she increasingly spoke to the analyst about her "little devil," letting herself go toward fantasies with anal content. Over time, this content began to manifest outside sessions as well, within the family – and especially at mealtime, which caused a certain degree of alarm in the parents.

Anna Freud considered that an error, which caused her to believe that she had transformed an inhibited and neurotic child into a "bad" child, and over the course of treatment, she herself took on the functions of the child's superego – in its dual aspects of prohibition and support, of restraining and of tolerating.

Melanie Klein

During those same years, Melanie Klein – who had been in analysis with Ferenczi and Abraham – on the basis of observations made of very small children, began experimenting in Berlin with a technique of interpreting play. This technique made great strides, especially when, after 1926, Klein moved to London. She emphasized the close relationship between the child's play and his psychosexual development. She had noticed a reduction in anxiety during the treatments, and that had confirmed her intuitions about the possibility of carrying out therapeutic treatments with very young children, utilizing direct interpretations regarding connections among play, fantasies, and the child's emotional conditions. The early phases of development became the object of deeper research, and to these she attributed an important meaning with respect to the way in which early object relationships came to be established. This led her to hypothesize that a nucleus of the superego's formation was already active well before what Freud had indicated, which connected it to the resolution of the oedipal complex. She saw the origin of subsequent psychic suffering in early anxieties and in the baby's depressive and paranoid experiences, and she dedicated herself to their cure by utilizing verbal interpretation and the transference, rejecting a pedagogical perspective in the child's therapy once she began to consider that his problems might be tied to the internal world, over which the parents had little influence in the present time.

In Klein's opinion, the superego or its early expression, relatively autonomous from the parents' influence – already present in the first year of life – was characterized by a fantasied severity that derived from the child's sadistic and cannibalistic impulses. Child analysis could thus set aside a pedagogical attitude, and in fact this came to be considered counterproductive, while through interpretations that approached deep contact with the mental contents of very young children, a reduction of anxiety was achieved. According to Klein, with children, too, transference to the analyst had to be taken into consideration from the beginning, as soon as psychopathological expressions were essentially linked to the configuration of the child's internal world.

It seems evident that these beliefs entered into competition with Freudian theories on the development of neurosis, in particular with Anna's, but at the same time it is undeniable that Kleinian contributions shone a bright light on the early phases of child development.

The confrontation did not end there. Two lines of research were created, two schools of thought, two formulations that have characterized the development of child analytic technique and its influence on the development of psychoanalytic thinking in general. Between the two women and between the two schools that then developed around Klein at the Tavistock Clinic and around Anna Freud at the

Hampstead Clinic (now the Anna Freud Centre), the controversies continued at length. They involved the British Psychoanalytical Society, which, thanks to the riveting theoretical confrontation that took place, received an exceptional boost to its research.

The climax of this debate, fraught with violent disputes and reciprocal accusations of "this isn't psychoanalysis," approached its zenith with a series of conferences to explore the various contributions, called the "Controversial Discussions," from 1942 to 1944. These discussions saw a total clash between the two lines of thinking.

Those years of acute conflict that, with ups and downs, has been dragged forward even to the present day, led to an agreement between "gentlewomen," which within the British Society took the form of a "third group." This third group tried to mediate the contrasting positions and to find a compromise with another great child psychoanalytic theoretician, Donald Winnicott, in a central position. Winnicott, a paediatrician who worked in a hospital, through his own personal journey that began from concrete knowledge of the child, began to explore important areas of the child's world, putting forward concepts such as that of holding, potential space, transitional phenomena, and play.

The Anna Freud School gave rise to ego psychology, which found broad acceptance most notably in North America, while the Kleinian theory of object relations had important influence primarily in Europe and Latin America. In this volume, one can find echoes of Winnicott's theoretical and clinical elaborations, as well as the voices of colleagues who come from both schools of thought.

One can trace the work of the Robertsons, who addressed the consequences of hospitalization, back to Anna Freud's ideas. Other contributions inspired by her work include Margaret Mahler's on the psychological birth of the infant and the journey toward separation-individuation in the early years of life; John Bowlby's on the theory of attachment; and current discussions on mentalization by Peter Fonagy and Mary Target.

Kleinian developments are recognized as an essential starting point for the work of Wilfred Bion, with the idea of the container-contained, the thinking apparatus, the concept of reverie, the alpha function, and group theory. In addition to Bion, I have frequently referenced in this book the work of Isabel Menzies Lyth and Elliott Jaques on institutions and their social models of protection against anxiety. I have also cited Esther Bick and her technique of infant observation, Donald Meltzer and his explorations of early autistic states, Antonino Ferro, Thomas Ogden, and James Grotstein.

One could say that Melanie Klein, Anna Freud and, to some degree Winnicott, drawing on their own individual characteristics, shed light on the areas of development highlighted by their personal history. Anna Freud turned to a child with more neurotic characteristics in which conflicts around management of instinctual impulses were played out, while Melanie Klein described a child with deeper areas of suffering, one in contact with psychotic areas of the personality. Winnicott was drawn to a child somewhat in the middle between the previous two, a child in whom – as in the borderline structures that he described – areas characterized by primitive anxieties could coexist with more developed areas.

Characteristics of Child Psychotherapy in Relation to Adult Psychotherapy

This schematic presentation of early theoretical positions in child analysis helps us understand the evolution that is taking place in this field and at the same time takes account of the complexity of material that, at a distance of almost a century, continues to have great relevance today. Since those early expositions, the positions of Anna Freud and Melanie Klein have been integrated, modified, and developed. Today the psychoanalyst does not exist who, once his training is behind him, does not make use of concepts (with more or less awareness) that stem from both these theoretical lines.

The rigid concept of neutrality is viewed with greater flexibility by Kleinians, while primary attention to the early phases of development is a common legacy for followers of Anna Freud. Furthermore, various attempts are in process that aim at emphasizing the clinical affinities of concepts expressed with different technical reference points. An example of this is the attempt to approach that complex interpsychic and intrapsychic dynamic that, through a complicated system of projected and identificatory mechanisms, gave rise to the Kleinian concept of projective identification and to others that can be grouped together with it, such as Anna Freud's concept of identification with the aggressor.

However, many things have changed in adult psychotherapy since that time, just as many have changed in child therapy. Child analysis is no longer concentrated on the search for hidden truth or on a hypothetical trauma but instead focuses on the flow of emotions between patient and therapist. In this way, the therapist can be helped to gain familiarity with those parts of himself that could not be accepted and to become more tolerant of wishes and fantasies that previously seemed inadmissible, thereby reducing the anxiety-provoking threat of conflicts with moral norms and reopening the way toward a personal developmental journey.

Differences in clinical approach between therapists of different schools of thought do not seem so important. From these various orientations, one can appreciate innovative aspects and overcome inadequate ones. At various meetings that address clinical material, the same language is often spoken.

Today when we speak of child psychotherapy, we do not mean only a process that is very closely tied to all the specific technical, logistical, and organizational conditions that make it possible (the setting), but with respect to an internal psychoanalytic framework, we mean the combination of technical interventions that allow adaptation of technique to the exigencies of the situation. That involves greater difficulties than in working with adults. For the child psychotherapist, it requires considerable flexibility, experience, ability, personal and theoretical training, and supervision – in order to determine the best ways and means to proceed with each individual case.

In contrast to adult therapy, which is not specifically indicated at moments of acute crisis (for example, when situations of grief, illness, or separation push the individual to concentrate all his resources and energies on a painful reality), in working with children, who often experience situations of crisis similar to those just mentioned, it is not possible to wait for those problems to be overcome, but instead it is important that one set out on a developmental course that in those problematic situations would otherwise risk being blocked. In discussing the subject of child psychotherapy, in fact, one cannot avoid addressing the concept of development, of growth.

With the adult, situations may be organized nosographically, to a degree, while in the child or adolescent, they assume very different meanings whenever one finds oneself dealing with a developmental accomplishment yet to take place, with structures not yet completely formed. The process of development is not linear. In order to grow, it is necessary to abandon modalities of psychic functioning that have been experienced as secure; there can be no development without the suffering tied to the changes that accompany transformations in ourselves and in our internal world. At an emotional level, the loss of a precariously balanced condition to attain a more satisfactory one implies the appearance of moments of difficulty that, once overcome, are transformed into elements of enrichment and maturation.

Early life phases are extraordinarily important. They require a physical and relational environment that enables the functions linked to emotional equilibrium to be solidified in a harmonious way and to be consolidated into a sense of affective security that forms the basis of all subsequent developments.

Psychosexual development, growing autonomy, and the complexity of intellectual development frequently pose problems for the child that have no easy solution. The ambivalence of the anal-sadistic phase and the coming to terms with aggressivity renew anxieties connected to very early life phases at a time when the process of separation-individuation must be defined. The birth of a little brother or sister added to this dynamic complicates it, causing new and more painful fears of separations, and it can lead to the appearance of regressive behaviours or various symptomatic expressions aimed at guaranteeing possession of the mother and the totality of her love.

The phallic phase, with its associated castration anxieties, the oedipal period, brings in the experience of a complicated loving relationship, with jealousies, rivalry, and inevitable frustrations. Adolescence – which, with the psychosomatic alterations of puberty, sets in motion a "second time" of the developmental trajectory of the early years of life, one in which the process of separation-individuation is defined with new challenges pertaining to sexual maturation and personal autonomy – constitutes another important moment at which an effective therapy can facilitate the evolution of obstacles and the overcoming of developmental breakdowns. These are sometimes transitory experiences, but they require considerable mental work to overcome – anxieties and difficulties – and they must be confronted by the child and by the adolescent in the course of the journey toward maturation.

But sometimes, it can happen that the child or adolescent is not in a condition to find adequate solutions or that the mother and father are not capable of completely fulfilling their parental function, of giving their son or daughter the help that s/he needs at a critical moment, and so the child is left to struggle with these problems alone. Moments of vulnerability can block the normal developmental process, accelerating it or derailing it through adaptive solutions that produce fault lines of pathology that can complicate the rest of life. In moments of this type, when the child's resources are not sufficient to cope with a developmental crisis, one offers appropriate therapeutic treatments that take on a preventative goal, beginning with the moment at which there is an attempt to identify early elements of suffering and the pathological mechanisms with which these elements are faced.

One of the objectives of a therapeutic intervention directed toward a still-growing subject is that of leading the patient into the channel of his developmental journey. The therapeutic goal consists of eliminating, as much as possible, repressions, interruptions, regressions, and conflicts in order to expand the ego's possibility of intervening, releasing the developmental forces so that they can continue to further the child's growth. To do this, it is necessary to be able to distinguish between those psychic disturbances that have been firmly constructed – where conflicts have been internalized and have involved ongoing modification of the internal world – and those psychic disturbances that have arisen due to missing elements in the external environment or to other factors that interfere with growth (serious family situations, illnesses, abandonments, organic or psychic deficits, etc.).

In conclusion, in returning to Giorgia and her problems, we can say that in her treatment, we see the goal of every psychoanalytic treatment, which is that of helping patients know and accept instinctual desires connected to the child part that exists in every human being and that may have given rise to conflicts and suffering. At times, a sort of "alphabetizing" of those parts exposed to early trauma may be required – parts that did not permit sensorial elements connected to the original trauma to gain access to a symbolic dimension. In these cases, the therapy tries to arrange for the patient to be able to tolerate the conflictual parts of the self that could reach psychic representation and, at the same time, not be forced to continually repeat in his/her behaviours the experiences connected to traumatic dimensions.

References

Freud, S. (1900). The interpretation of dreams. *S. E.*, 1/2.

———. (1905). Three essays on the theory of sexuality. *S. E.*, 7.

———. (1908). Analysis of a phobia in a five-year-old boy ("Little Hans"). *S. E.*, 10.

Grosskurth, P. (1986). *Melanie Klein: Her World and Her Work*. Northvale, NJ/London: Jason Aronson, 1995.

Misès, R. & Quemada, N. (2002). La classification française des troubles mentaux de l'enfant et de l'adolescent: présentation générale. *Annales Médico-psychologiques, Revue Psychiatrique*, 160:210–212.

Winnicott, D. W. (1965). *The Maturational Processes and the Facilitating Environment.* London: Routledge, 2018.

Chapter 6

A Child Psychoanalytic Treatment

The Irish Sky

In the course of treatment with a child whom I will call Daniele, a popular song often came to mind. The song was about the Irish sky that always accompanies a person and allows him to dance with gypsies and kings; this song often popped into my mind, for various reasons. First, because Ireland was one of the places that, in Daniele's fantasies, we had visited many times during the course of our meetings. Then too, the music and the dance represented a kind of soundtrack, a means of expressing the emotional content that was at first hidden and then became more understandable. And last, because the Irish sky made me think of the narcissistic foundation that allows us to face the complexity of life, to dance with gypsies or kings – something that Daniele seemed capable of doing at the end of treatment, leaving behind his solitary ways in which he had been deprived of dancing.

I began seeing Daniele when, at seven years of age, he was brought to me because of a deep disturbance in relationships, academic difficulties, and very bizarre behaviours. He was the eldest child in his family, with a brother a year-and-a-half younger. He often lived in a world all his own, frequently immersed in dialogue with an imaginary friend, and he responded to requests made to him by repeating the question.

Continually in frenetic motion, Daniele loved to express himself by interpreting the role of a musical pop star, either a man or frequently a woman, through dances and songs that formed a solipsistic and repetitive performance, of which he was the sole protagonist. This was a performance that couldn't be shared with other children, whom he tried to involve but to whom he left only the role of spectators. His way of singing was peculiar, bringing to mind a "one-man band" – the street musicians who sing and play various instruments at the same time. His instruments with which to keep time were his mouth, tongue, and lips, which in various highly idiosyncratic ways he would click or smack to form a basic rhythm, into which he inserted the words and melodies of his songs that he followed as he danced.

Daniele's parents, both professionals who were very busy and dedicated to their jobs, described a great struggle to remain in contact with him. From the time that he was very little, Daniele had been entrusted to his grandparents and a babysitter

DOI: 10.4324/9781003252238-7

because his mother had resumed working almost full-time when he was three months old. The early separation from his mother seemed to be capped by a poor relationship and sudden separation from a babysitter when he was six or seven months old. The parents said that they had had to let this babysitter go when they realized that something wasn't going well between her and Daniele; whenever he saw her, he would start to cry, trying to hide behind his mother.

After some months of observation, in which disturbed relationships tinged by hysterical traits were evident, I initiated therapy at a frequency of two sessions per week, moving on to three weekly sessions after almost a year; altogether his treatment lasted four years.

The relationship between us began in a very intense way and continued in a similar vein over the course of treatment, vacillating between various positive and negative, narcissistic and object-related gradations in the transference; that is, a mixture was transposed onto the analyst of the emotions and affects sequentially felt by the patient toward significant persons of his past.

A lengthy early period was dedicated to establishing a relationship with a child who required me to take part as a spectator who listened to his songs and witnessed his little dances. I tried to intervene verbally, with little result, when it seemed appropriate – especially by setting limits when his movements became dangerous, such as when he got up onto tables, climbed into cupboards, or left the consulting room for long periods of time, trying to explore all areas of my office suite. I had to lock the private rooms of my office area, leaving open only the door to the bathroom, another location where he often took refuge for long periods.

From the beginning, like a narcissistic double of himself, he imagined living with me in a city called "Catia," which would then become Ireland, or part of a Finland that diverged from the Apennines, including the Alps and extending into northern Europe. Beyond having a world of our own, we also had our own time, where months and days of the week were not the conventional ones but had an alphabetical or numerical order.

At the beginning, his way of playing was barely sketched out. He tended to take over the entire contents of the toy box, rapidly using all the paper, crayons, and games in a way that wasn't very constructive, asking me only to follow him in his play and to replenish materials as he used them up.

He soon told me that he found the world

> 100% difficult. For me the world seems to be a trap, a trap in hell. There are some bad people who treat others badly, who make fun of them. I can't live like that. You never see calm people; they just go around looking lost. And they tell me I'm crazy! The earth is awful, I hate it, I hope that it dies. If people are like this, I can't deal with them. In soccer, where I haven't wanted to go any more because it's a terrible game, they told me I have a shit-name. At catechism they asked me why I don't wear shorter pants. At the gym they called me a faggot, and I don't even know what that means. Life is good when children are very small; the life of school-age children is unbearable.

From our initial sessions, Daniele made it clear that our meetings represented for him a very important moment. I felt myself to be fulfilling the role of a basic object for him but also that he felt he had to keep me under constant control. I was important and dangerous, primarily loved but not exclusively so; under his appealing surface, little aggressive acts appeared, such as secretly breaking off the leaves of a plant in my office.

In his stories, an internal world emerged that had both idealized good parts and very dangerous bad parts:

> There are parents who want to be alone and exclude their children – very bad moms who impose punishments on children for a period of 10,000 weeks, or who have stolen and been sent to prison, and dads who lose patience.

In one of his stories that unfolded in a place called Catia, while using puppets to enact a scene of family life, Daniele suddenly threw all the puppets into the air, launching them violently against a wall. He said: "An earthquake occurred. And when there's an earthquake, little houses with no strength fall down."

In the next session as well, he proposed playing in Catia, where the dad, son, and daughter were going to a concert. The mom was in prison, and when I asked Daniele why, he said that she would be there one or two days because she had left her child alone. He told me that long ago, Catia had been a very beautiful city, but then there was a very serious earthquake, the strongest earthquake in all the world. Referring to the transference relationship via the word "tree" (*albero* in Italian) – which for some patients calls to mind my last name because of its sound – he told me that all Catia had been destroyed and not a single tree remained. Luckily, the toy tree that he was playing with was in New York; otherwise it, too, would have died.

It seemed to me that in this session, Daniele brought to life various dimensions of his relationship with the object; for example, rage for the delinquent mom who had left her child alone covered a traumatic rupture of the primary relationship that he re-enacted, excitedly mastering it. He tried to rescue me from this destructiveness, keeping me alive, leaving me on the edges of the conversation, thereby protecting me from a connection to him that he felt was too intense – both for its destructiveness and its sexual excitement.

After a break for the first summer vacation, while obsessive ideas were present – "I want everything beautiful, everything clean" – themes connected with anality appeared with greater frequency. He played at selling precious things, such as gold rings and other jewellery that he constructed with play objects, and when he found small, antiquated objects in boxes, these became excrement.

Daniele struggled to tell me that he felt others had it in for him because he always made mistakes – even his friends, who never invited him to play with them. He then spoke of the brother who slept with their parents, but this thought quickly became too painful and he needed to detach, changing the subject and singing in a very high voice – which for him represented both a way of expressing sad thoughts and at the same time evacuating them.

Two families appeared in his play: a lively one, welcoming and calm, and a second one that was easily irritated and was characterized by nervous and aggressive movements. In one session, the mom suddenly fell into a well and called for help – which was denied her because she was bad. She was a mom who, with sudden movements, sent away her children, and Daniele then broke up everything, threw it all into the air, even the little table on which we were working – as though intense suffering, a sudden impulse, had brought him to the destruction of thinking.

More than a year after the therapy began – with sessions characterized by my adaptation to the patient's needs, and without much possibility of inserting myself into his fantasies except in the very rare moments when he almost allowed me to – he began to accept more of my perspectives and my more active presence in the session. More and more, I noticed that if the expression of aggressivity, of sexual excitement and authentic drive manifestations seemed to constitute a danger that led him to fear a rupture in a precarious narcissistic balance, the control of the other, often exercised with a sort of excitation, seemed at times to represent a cage that imprisoned him.

Thus, an idea gradually began to take shape in my mind: that alongside a deprived child who demanded to be listened to and cared for, there was a child with neurotic characteristics, excited and overbearing, who by employing a castling strategy in his defensive system could checkmate the world.

Eric Brenman (1999) states that in the hysterical character, with its characteristics of splitting and projection, there is a combination of catastrophe and denial: "The patient is persecuted by objects to which he attributes a great number of atrocious, catastrophic stories . . . while the remaining part of the personality seems to function well" (p. 218, translation by G. Atkinson).

Brenman emphasizes the narcissistic use that the hysteric makes of the external object, who is apparently "utilized" as an internal object with which to attack him and subjugate him in his psychic reality. This occurs because an internal relationship about which the subject can articulate ambivalence would expose him to a renewed experience of catastrophe. This information was useful to me in finding meaning in the transference to my being important to Daniele, while at the same time I was denied my individual reality.

Anne Alvarez (2016) and Angelo Macchia (2015) write that the experience with patients of this type may lead the analyst to ask himself questions about his own transferential experience and to shift from a phase of support/caregiving (of a "maternal" type) to a phase of confrontation-interpretation (more of a "paternal" type).

Semi (1995) writes of an implicit risk in relationships with patients with hysterical traits, referring to the complex system of identifications that involve the analyst and his narcissism. In deep unconscious contact with the patient, there can be an identification with parts of him by means of a hysterical identification through which "the subject is identified with an aspect, a detail, a complex, a wish, an unconscious drive motion of the other" (p. 245, translation by G. Atkinson).

My having understood that my own narcissism was also at play and was leading me to principally focus on the deprived child instead of the child who was embroiled in a more developed conflict (though an underground one) took shape at a countertransferential level in my recognized need to "extricate" myself from the role that Daniele had assigned to me. I was thus led to keep in mind, with tact and sensitivity, others of his (and my) narcissistic needs – even his violent excitation and his libidinal investment in me.

At about that time, the "story" took shape – a narrative connected to early traumatic experiences that we would then often refer to when we looked for words with which to describe sensorial experiences connected to the loss of a relationship, a collapse that happened some time earlier, tied to a maternal incapacity that left him prey to intense anxieties.

The "story" became more and more important because it allowed Daniele to gain some distance from the "real" pressure of his anxieties, since "it's not completely done yet." With great pain, he related a fantasy in which everyone was angry with him and threw him into a very deep canyon. Over time this theme was enriched by variations, some of which were also positive, such as one in which he got married and had a family.

Three Sessions After the Second Summer Vacation

At the first session after the second summer break since he had begun seeing me, Daniele, crying desperately, immediately began to tell me about his difficulty responding to his family's and his school's expectations. It was almost as though he were imploring of me, "I'm not asking you to do impossible things, but do what you can to help me." This session, with the degree of suffering that Daniele expressed and that he was able to link to my absence over the summer, reinforced for me the possibility of proposing to his family the shift to three weekly sessions that I had had in mind for some time. The family accepted this proposal, and with the switch to three sessions, our way of working changed radically, especially in regard to the possibility of interventions in the transference dimension.

A couple of months later, having begun the session with a restrained tone and keeping himself distant in the conversation, Daniele asked me what the origin of my last name was.

While speaking, he tied his shoes, resting his feet on the little table on which we worked. Confirming the aggressive and transgressive quality of that gesture, he farted and said to me: "Sorry, it just slipped out! I have to go to the bathroom!" Somewhat jokingly, he said, "Oh gosh, now you're mad at me." He went to the bathroom and washed his hands, continuing to say to me from behind the door, "Sorry, it just slipped out."

After some minutes, he returned to the office and asked me what time "this place" closed, and where did I go afterward. "I want to know what your day is like," he said, sitting in the armchair behind the desk, facing drawers that were not perfectly closed, and added with a tone of reproof: "You always forget to close the drawers!"

"You wake up at 8:30," he continued,

> and then you go to Sant'Orsola Hospital until 1:00. Then you eat. Then you resume working, and at 4:45 you come here and we play until 5:30. Then somebody arrives; the two of you talk and talk and talk. Or maybe before that there's someone else. Then at 7:30, you go home and eat.

I answered that maybe he thought that, if I were with someone else, what he believed had happened with his mother could happen here – that he was afraid of being abandoned, thrown away.

In response he made another stink. I then told him that a doctor who neglected him and who was with other people deserved a stink. Daniele said, "Yes – are you mad? Are you going to throw me out?"

In that moment, I recalled that in the previous session, with no apparent reaction on his part, I had communicated that the next week I would have to skip a session. So I then said that my upcoming absence might make him feel neglected and not very important. Daniele said, "It's true – I thought it must be an appointment so important that you can't forget it" (here he used *forget* to mean *change*). "I think that this appointment must be very important if you prefer it to me, and so I don't feel accepted, welcomed."

I said: "So perhaps you thought: 'I won't say anything to the doctor, and in fact I'll make the stink that he deserves.'"

Daniele said: "No, it's not true – you're making fun of me! In our world, people are not made fun of." Immediately after this remark, he began to dance and sing, and for a while he made me watch one of his performances, one in which a woman was teetering inside a canyon.

It seemed that Daniele had finally expressed with greater clarity an oscillation between various states of psychic organization – between an ego with more precarious functioning in which narcissistic/identity-related problems appeared to dominate and a relatively high-functioning ego that saw the importance of sexuality – of bisexuality – and that returned to the scene in the form of a hysterical configuration.

Green (1997) mentions a continuity between hysteria and borderline cases, and his observations have been useful to me in attempting to give a sense of coherent meaning to what I was experiencing in my work with Daniele. According to Green, in borderline cases, the ego's fragility harkens back to early trauma and to early maternal influence, to the fear of being at the mercy of an omnipotent object: "In hysteria, conflicts connected to erotic aspects of the psyche predominate, while in borderline cases, it is destructivity that is in the foreground and that tends to distort or cover over the erotic problem" (1997, p. 346; translation by G. Atkinson).

Some Months After the Third Interruption for Summer Vacation

I thought that Daniele was capable of being present at one of the two annual meetings that I would typically have with his parents. It seemed to me that this would be useful, especially so that he would not have the feeling that something was happening between the adults that he didn't know about. The meeting was not especially problematic; there was an exchange between the parents' point of view and Daniele's. My attitude was one of listening and facilitation of the encounter, but the consequences of what that meeting meant to Daniele would require many meetings in order to be fully expressed.

Three weeks later, after a period in which Daniele expressed resentment and disdain for "disgusting" Tuscany (his paternal family's region), as well as his love for the beauty and sweetness of Liguria (his mother's region), he began his session by complaining and crying. "You forgot something important – you didn't tell me – you shouldn't forget, and if you do, you don't have our presence together at heart," he complained, causing me to recall that I had not referred to the fact that several days earlier, I had had a birthday, which he knew fell within that period. A lengthy early part of the session saw him crying and shouting at my assumed forgetfulness and the fact that we could not celebrate the event together.

I vacillated between authentically feeling Daniele's displeasure at not being considered important enough to me and the awareness that my "omission" allowed him to express negative transference elements that had come to light in recent sessions. Referring to moments of intense rage in the previous session, I told him that, in effect, last time had led me to see that he was somewhat angry with me. After a little while, Daniele calmed down, continually resorting to a musical rhythm that absorbed his attention. Then, after I told him that at any rate, I found it important that he had made me understand what he felt, he answered, almost shouting: "Okay, I forgive you, but you must have a penance! You have to write that the Tuscany of the Filippi family [a made-up name] is full of crap. The Filippis are idiots and Tuscany is awful."

I commented that today, too, I didn't seem to be behaving well. He said:

Albertone [he had creatively manipulated my last name to come up with "Big Albert"], today you violated the work of the important genius Daniele, head of Ireland. Albertone has been very bad and has been stupid lately, really stupid! And Daniele is very angry with him because he had promised to tell him when his birthday got here. Now Daniele has pardoned him, but Albertone must pay attention because it's a "violation" of our work in Ireland – because if you do something "in violation" next time, you'll get a bigger punishment.

I said:

But this time, Daniele was afraid to tell Albertone that he had made him angry because he thought that Albertone wouldn't want to be with him any more and would make him fall into the canyon, like in the story. And so as not to let him know how angry he was, Daniele talked to Albertone about Tuscany and the Filippis because Albertone, like his dad, had really made him angry.

Daniele replied, "For now, Albertone is in the Tuscany of the Filippis, of the bad people, while before he was in the Liguria of the Visco family [another made-up name], with the good people."

"Certainly, Daniele is happy to have found a way to be close to his mom and to feel that his mom loves him," I said. "And because of this, certain people, like Renzo Filippi [his dad], are better off sent to that horrid Tuscany with Albertone."

Daniele laughed heartily at my observations. I emphasized that he seemed happy we could finally talk and laugh about these things. He said that next time, I would have to undergo what he called a "Blue Ray interrogation test of the work we've done this year." (I imagine that he took the term "Blue Ray" from high-quality DVD technology.) If I passed the test, I could go back to Liguria with the good Visco family, with Daniele; otherwise I would have to stay with the disgusting Tuscans. Daniele said, "There are twenty questions – you'll certainly do it, you can answer them. My brother is in Tuscany too because he's just like Dad, because he's bad."

At the next session, Daniele immediately proposed the "Blue Ray Testimonial" that he had promised me, with which I could earn the right to return to Liguria and be with him and his mother. (I thought of the "penances" in the games of my childhood: "To say, to do, to kiss, letter, testimonial.") I learned that there would be some questions, six in all, to which I would have to reply.

Then Daniele took my notebook and wrote down the first question: "What was the first city that we used in our play?" I answered by writing, "Catia." "Very good," he commented, giving me a 10.

The second question was: "Our country where we lived in this game was–?" I wrote, "Ireland," and earned another compliment and another 10.

The third was: "Outside, were there fruits or vegetables?" Here I was a little less brilliant and earned a 9.

The fourth was:

The 'media' story – is it the one about engaging a nice and peaceful life? Or about my brother's wedding, where everyone has a girlfriend and I don't? Or the one where my whole family wants to kill me and makes me fall into a canyon of fire with my mom, who falls in headlong with my grandmother and my other grandmother?

Here he got a little confused in his handwriting, but when I answered that the "media" was the second one, he was quite satisfied and gave me another 10.

Question #5: "The days and seasons of Old Ireland – how were they ordered, alphabetically or in real order?" I answered that they were in alphabetical order, and I got another 10.

The sixth question was oral rather than written, and to my great surprise, Daniele asked me how many times he had cried in sessions since we resumed after the summer break. He said that there were two times, and he wanted me to list them. I told him I thought he had once cried because he couldn't do his homework and he feared he couldn't succeed at being a boy like other boys. On the other occasion, it seemed to me that he cried because he had the impression his mother was making fun of him. I also said I thought he had cried more on this second occasion.

This last question was worth 11 points, and Daniele was very happy to give me an overall score of 60, the highest grade. He congratulated me and said that I had won, and that I could now go back to the Liguria of the good people.

I marvelled at the way that, through these questions, he had showed me that he was keeping the contents of our sessions perfectly in mind, since their beginning. However, he wanted to know whether I kept him in my mind as well and if he could trust me – whether our relationship could support negative transference elements and whether in my mind there was room for a child who felt emotions and contradictory feelings toward me, similar to those he felt toward his parents. Catia, Ireland, and Finland were not only places in the mind in which to keep positive things, but they could also host feelings of hostility that until then he had had to keep out of our relationship, due to worry that the feared catastrophe would take place and that the story could still come to life.

Elements of Passage

In many other sessions, I experienced in the relationship with Daniele what Winnicott (1962) says about the existence of two mothers for the child, the *mother-object* and the *mother-environment*. Although Daniele, under the pressure of intense drive conflictuality, attacked the mother-object part of me, in our relationship he also experienced my function of mother-environment in providing a sort of para-excitatory/protective filter with regard to the intensity of the emotions he felt.

In many sessions, Daniele arrived with a darkened face and stretched out on an armchair huddling down or moved around the room restlessly. He shouted at length, sometimes at the top of his voice – or at times in a more contained tone – an anguished "Come on! Come on! Come on!"

This exhortation/imploring transmitted a sense of profound desperation and seemed to carry sensory elements connected to the relationship with a primary object. In those moments, my words had no effect; on some occasions, he listened to what he himself said, to the sounds he produced, or even the noise of air passing through his throat. At those times, which made me think of autistic states, he sometimes added bodily movements, such as licking his lips in a circular way, an area implied in the movement of suction during nursing, as though he wanted to call to mind memories of the body (Gaddini 1981) – almost to feel its borders, the surface that separates inside from outside.

Invariably, in the course of every session, after a period of variable length in which he was absorbed in private fantasies, little by little Daniele began to create a melody, a singsong in which he seemed completely absorbed. This would start with movements of his lips and mouth, from which he slowly made a rhythm emerge, as well as words through which he tried to communicate what he was thinking. Depending on how he felt, this could last rather a long time, sometimes for most of the session, though he set aside some time at the end to recompose himself, often seated near me or huddling down on my legs to then reassure me, saying he wasn't angry with me, and in turn wanting reassurance that I was not angry with him. When he greeted the family member who came to pick him up, he did not betray any trace of the violent sensations he had expressed in the session.

In the course of Daniele's sessions, in the alternation between various moments that I have described and that often caused me trepidation about his capacity to be in contact with reality and about my own capacity to be in contact with such an intense and piercing pain, I often asked myself how the regulatory structures come into being – the narcissistic basis that forms the background of an individual's emotional security.

The suffering that Daniele expressed seemed to me to be rooted in the earliest experiences of the formation of the self, when the object is primarily lived as the environment, not separated or distinct from the child, before the mother becomes an object perceived subjectively in the not-me space. The position that Ogden (1989) defines *contiguous-autistic*, from the earliest phases of life, "under normal circumstances can be seen to provide the bounded sensory 'floor' . . . of experience" (p. 45).

> The normal elaboration of the contiguous-autistic organization depends upon the capacity of the mother and infant to generate forms of sensory experience that "heal" or "make bearable" the awareness of the separateness that is an intrinsic component of early infantile experience.
>
> [Ogden 1989, pp. 51–52]

In my opinion, what saved Daniele from more massive emotional withdrawal was the experience, at some level, of an intense contact that he perceived in the connection, before the rupture. Certain object investments – always precarious, always at risk of interruption, but at any rate experienced and able to activate his fantasy life and drive investments – allowed him to remain in the area of neurosis.

Conclusion

I left Daniele when he attended the second year of middle school. His scholastic performance was sufficient, and his relationships with companions were difficult but in a positive way, without the criticality of earlier years. In his relationship with me as well, there were no more peaks of suffering or disagreement that he had expressed during our early years of therapy. Peaceful sessions were mixed with sessions in which he talked to me about his difficulties in an emotional tone far removed from the anxious one that I have tried to describe in this chapter. Obsessive symptomatology was still present, but with less intense manifestations. Often the sessions left me with the feeling of an enjoyable relationship with a child who was doing well.

After a good summer vacation, the fourth since we started working together, Daniele resumed his sessions with an air of "home sweet home." In one session during the final period, in which I had the sensation of being with a child like any other, he said to me, "Write," as he did every time he had the feeling of telling me something important. And he dictated:

> I have painful times, crying that I can't stand, and sometimes when I come here, let's say about once in three months, it is the best day of the year, and the unburdening of what I feel and the crying go away. The things that we do here are what explodes in rage and then becomes beautiful.

On another occasion, almost to emphasize the introjection of analytic functions he had achieved, Daniele said to me:

> I don't like paper because as soon as you touch it, it's ruined, and I also don't like electronic objects like iPhones because they break. A tree [*albero*/D'Alberton] doesn't break; even if a tree is hit and only part of it remains, it then heals, and in the end maybe even the scar is gone. The tree resists.

References

Alvarez, A. (2016). Vari tipi di depressione: lo stato degli oggetti interni [Various types of depression: The state of internal objects]. Paper presented at Bologna Psychoanalytic Center, January 23.

Brenman, E. (1999). Isteria [Hysteria]. In *Perché l'isteria? Attualità di una malattia ontologica [Why Hysteria? Current Viewpoints on an Ontological Illness]*, ed. F. Scalzone & G. Zontini. Naples, Italy: Ligouri.

Gaddini, E. (1981). Early defensive fantasies and the psychoanalytical process. In *A Psychoanalytic Theory of Infantile Experience: Conceptual and Clinical Reflections*, ed. A. Limentani. London: Institute of Psychoanalysis, 1992.

Green, A. (1997). Il chiasma: i casi limiti visti dalla prospettiva dell'isteria, l'isteria vista retrospettivamente a partire dai casi limiti [Chiasmus: Prospective – borderlines viewed after hysteria; retrospective – hysteria viewed after borderlines (part I)]. In *Perché l'isteria? Attualità di una malattia ontologica [Why Hysteria? Current Viewpoints on an Ontological Illness]*, ed. F. Scalzone & G. Zontini. Naples, Italy: Ligouri. Also in *Bulletin, European Psychoanalytical Federation*, pp. 28–45, July 3.

Macchia, A. (2015). Verso l'(O)rigine della relazione analitica [On the foundation of the analytic relationship]. Paper given at Bologna Psychoanalytic Center, October 22.

Ogden, T. H. (1989). *The Primitive Edge of Experience*. Lanham, NJ: Jason Aronson/Rowman & Littlefield, 1992.

Semi, A. A. (1995). Sull'Isteria e sull'identificazione isterica [On hysteria and hysterical identification]. *Rivista di Psicoanalisi*, 41:237–254.

Winnicott, D. W. (1962). The development of the capacity for concern. In *The Maturational Processes and the Facilitating Environment*, ed. D. W. Winnicott. London: Routledge, 2018.

Chapter 7

Therapeutic Consultations with Parents of Young Children

What sorrow has come upon your heart?
Speak out; hide it not in your mind, that we both may know.

[Homer, *The Iliad*, Book 1, line 345]

Almost on its own, interest in parent-child psychotherapeutic consultations has inserted itself into my observations about my professional practice. This interest has been reinforced by my hospital work, beginning with the formidable tool represented by the paediatric hospital and the extraordinary opportunity to capture expressions of emotional discomfort that in the early years of life are expressed primarily through the body.

In working with the parents of small children in various contexts, I noticed empirically how much influence even a single meeting could sometimes have in resolving difficulties in the relationship that are expressed via the usual symptoms of early childhood: primarily disturbances of eating, sleeping, attachment, or early behaviour. Alongside situations that require longer, more structured interventions, I was astonished by the rapidity of changes that took place in some cases. By contrast, in many case histories of children and adolescents, one could see how a request for help that had not been honoured in early childhood may still be an unsettled score after some years, especially in early adolescence. In this period, in fact, the stimulus of puberty and the new iteration of the separation-individuation process – which leads the child to become even more differentiated from the mother and to be capable of engaging in activities for somewhat longer periods of time without the parents' presence (Mahler et al. 1975; Pellizzari 2009) – can reactivate old traumatic fault lines (D'Alberton 2016).

In the past 40 years, parent and child consultations have been the object of growing interest from paediatricians, psychoanalysts, and child psychotherapists. In various parts of the world, different experiences have taken place that, together with theoretical and territorial specificity, demonstrate important elements of affinity (Bruno and Norsa 2009; Cena et al. 2010; Magnini and Sala 2013).

DOI: 10.4324/9781003252238-8

In reality, from a clinical point of view, a relationship between parental problems and children's physical and psychological conditions had already been described since the dawn of psychoanalysis. In one of the early "pre-analytic" cases recounted in "A Case of Successful Treatment by Hypnotism" (1892–1893), Freud was called in to intervene with a young mother who, although she wanted to breastfeed her baby, was not capable of it. She did not have enough milk, and she suffered during breastfeeding; she had lost her appetite and couldn't sleep. Entrusting the baby to a wet nurse seemed to resolve the situation for both baby and mother.

The young Freud intervened again three years later when a second baby was born and the mother had the same problem in trying to breastfeed the new arrival. Freud conducted two sessions of hypnosis that seemed to resolve things:

> She had an excellent appetite and plenty of milk for the baby, there was not the slightest difficulty when it was put to her breast, and so on. . . . The mother fed her child for eight months, and I had many opportunities of satisfying myself in a friendly way that they were both doing well.
>
> [Freud 1892–1893, p. 120]

The treatments during that period were brief by nature and incorporated a certain level of activity on the part of the therapist, who utilized hypnosis, suggestion, and advice of various types that today we would tend to avoid. Freud himself – in a note written 30 years later – recognized that "no analyst can read this case history to-day without a smile of pity" (Freud 1893, p. 105; footnote added in 1924).

He had not yet encountered the "40-year-old from Livonia" (Freud 1893), the baroness Emmy von N., whose treatment contributed to subsequent modifications of technique and in whose case a line of transgenerational suffering seems to be defined with greater clarity. Next to the last in a series of siblings of whom only four were living, Emmy von N. had a childhood marked by episodes of mourning. "She was brought up carefully, but under strict discipline by an over-energetic and severe mother" (Freud 1893, p. 49), and the mother, too, died when Emmy was 19 years old.

At 23, she married a man much older than she with whom she had two daughters. He died of a cardiac problem while Emmy was sick in bed after the birth of her second-born; she found herself feeling hostile toward this daughter, attributing to the baby the responsibility for her illness and her husband's death, since in having to stay close to the baby she hadn't been able to take care of him. A few weeks later, the baby began to exhibit extreme restlessness, sleep disturbances, and an important developmental deterioration.

This clinical case is important because it forced Freud to modify his working method when, in facing some of his insistent questions, the mother burst out "in a definitely grumbling tone that I was not to keep on asking her where this and that came from, but to let her tell me what she had to say" (Freud 1893, p. 63). Rather reluctantly, Freud agreed, and suddenly he surprised himself by thinking that the conversation with the baroness was not

> so aimless as would appear. On the contrary, it contains a fairly complete reproduction of the memories and new impressions which have affected her since our last talk, and it often leads on, in a quite unexpected way, to patho- genic reminiscences of which she unburdens herself without being asked to. It is as though she had adopted my procedure and was making use of our conversation, apparently unconstrained.
>
> [p. 56]

The method of free association had come to light, and from then on overly active attitudes on the analyst's part were gradually abandoned. This attitude, with the distance of some years, came to be reinforced by the concept of evenly sus- pended attention.

> Experience soon showed that the attitude which the analytic physician could most advantageously adopt was to surrender himself to his own unconscious mental activity, in a state of evenly suspended attention, to avoid so far as possible reflection and the construction of conscious expectations, not to try to fix anything that he heard particularly in his memory, and by these means to catch the drift of the patient's unconscious with his own unconscious.
>
> [Freud 1923, p. 239]

Historical Trends in Parent-child Treatments

In the vignettes from the prehistory of psychoanalysis that have just been cited, some factors are already present that subsequent research would identify as able to influence the parent-child relationship. For example, when a child, invested with both love and aggressivity, finds himself the depository of traits that the par- ents don't recognize in themselves, such as occurred for Emmy von N.'s daughter, she renews the connection with a lost object in the mother's personal history, the husband, toward whom mourning has not been elaborated.

Despite the enormous differences that separate us from those times, certain characteristics are evident that strike us today as well when we encounter parents who find themselves coping with the difficulties of a young child, and after having spoken with a paediatrician, they accept the option of consulting a therapist. In these consultations, something astonishing frequently happens, with such radical and quick changes that one thinks of the power of suggestion, even though long- term work is often required to reinforce the gains and to avoid new problems that present at later points in life.

After Freud, it was Ferenczi who added missing elements in the early envi- ronment to the field of observation – the "pre-primal (*ururtraumatisch*) trauma mother-child scar" (1932, p. 83) and its influence in determining a multiform traumatic dimension, the expression of early mother-child phantasms and of the parents' fantasies about their children. In later times, Abraham and Torok (1978) spoke of transgenerational transmission of the parents' unconscious fantasies and of familial phantasms through a "hidden and imaginary identification" (p. 292) with unthought areas, denied and expelled by the other. Aulagnier (1975) underlined the possible presence, alongside a word that supports and accepts, of a word that can violate the child's subjectivity. Faimberg (2005) described identifications transferred through unconscious fantasies – mentally unrepresented and unrepresentable – in the parents, passed from one generation to another. Bollas (1987) devoted attention to mining and setting aside identifications that were products of the child's interiorization of the parents' reasoning and their unconscious fantasies.

Parent-child consultations, as we now understand them, came into being in the public sphere as a theoretical-ideological option that originated with the clinical necessity of reducing the duration of treatment, in order to be able to provide answers to a greater number of patients compared to those who could be treated by psychoanalysts. The format of these consultations was derived from brief psychotherapy for adults centred on a particular problem (Cramer and Palacio Espasa 1993; Stern 1995). After the first essentially orthodox attempts during the pioneering phase (Ferenczi and Rank 1923), the second generation of analysts tried to define briefer forms of psychotherapy, narrowing the focus – the patient's "zone of conflict" – on which to concentrate the therapeutic work (Alexander and French 1946; Balint 1957). Starting in the 1960s, these attempts were again taken up by Malan, Sifneos, and Davanloo (see Migone 2004).

In the paediatric field, Winnicott (1965), with his extensive hospital experience, dedicated careful attention to psychotherapeutic meetings with parents or children that, although essentially diagnostic, for him also took on a therapeutic tone. While not defining his technique as "psychoanalysis," he maintained that considerable experience in clinical psychoanalytic practice was required in order to put it into practice. He first addressed himself to the person who presented as the patient; sometimes he did not even see the parents. He maintained that the first meetings had a basic importance, since in analysis, "the first interview may be reduplicated, or may be extended as an 'on demand therapy' over months or even years" (Winnicott 1971, p. 306).

Winnicott's basic principle was to offer "a humane setting" in which the therapist allowed the person consulting him to utilize the space of the consultation as he believed would be best: "The therapist will not distort the course of events, doing or not doing things based on his own anxiety or on his sense of guilt or his need to achieve success" (1965, p. 345, translation by G. Atkinson).

But it was the intense period of French-speaking child psychiatry during the Second World War that caused early childhood to become the fulcrum and centre of interest in therapeutic consultations that drew on psychoanalysis, as seen in the work of Kreisler et al. (1974), Lebovici et al. (1985), Kreisler (1981), de Ajuriaguerra (1993), Françoise Dolto (1971, 1985), and Didier Houzel (2010). Today as well, it is possible to make use of this fertile cultural tradition through the creative contributions of Bernard Golse (2006) and his work at Necker Hospital in Paris, of Sylvain Missonier with perinatal consultation (2003), of Marie José Soubieux and Michel Soulé with foetal consultation (2005), and of Anne Marie Moro with transcultural consultations (1994).

In England, various experiences were taking shape, primarily at the "Under Five Counseling Center" in Tavistock (Miller 1994) and the Anna Freud Centre in London, where research was developed on transgenerational transmission of attachment patterns (Fonagy and Target 1997), which utilized concepts of transmission of internal operative models and of the development of the reflective function of the self to suggest interventions based on mentalization – that is, the capacity to imagine mental states in the self and in others.

Almost all authors interested in disturbances of early childhood have noted the importance, in both therapeutic and preventative terms, of early instances of taking into account problems in the relationship between parents and children. The assumption is that the younger the child, the less his internal world has been structured, and his personality organization is more elastic and sensitive to interactions with parents.

Working in the paediatric arena, in fact, one has occasion to notice that requests for consultation about issues connected to the body but rooted in the emotional dimension, as well as in the relationship with parents, centre primarily on two especially important periods in life: early childhood and early adolescence. It is as though in early childhood the basis is laid down on which subsequent psychic development depends, and puberty represents a way to test the solidity of narcissistic supportive structures established in the first years of life.

This is an additional motive, then, to devote attention to factors that not only allow intervening on a criticality in action but also to fulfil a preventative function for the future.

Data from the Neurosciences

By now there is universal recognition of the importance of early relationships in determining an individual's emotional, affective, and cognitive competency.

> Experiences in the earliest years of life form the foundation of brain architecture, for better or for worse. Learning, behavior, and health across the lifespan are all built on that foundation.
> [Center on the Developing Child, Harvard University; http://developingchild.harvard.edu/resources/ from-best-practices-to-breakthrough-impacts/]

From this same group of researchers, we learn that neural connections for sensory pathways of vision and hearing, of language and higher cognitive functions, reach their maximal level within the first year of life. The prenatal and early postnatal period is in fact characterized by a hyperbolic proliferation in sequence and an overproduction of the number of synapses, under the control of the genes activated by experiences.

> At its peak, some 15,000 synapses are produced on every cortical neuron, which corresponds to a rate of 1.8 million new synapses *per second* between two months of gestation and two years after birth!
>
> [Eliot 1999, p. 27, emphasis in original]

> In the first few years of life, each neuron forms about 15,000 synapses. By the age of 2, the child has as many synapses as an adult, and by age 3 this has doubled to about 1,000 trillion. This number holds through a lot of shuffling about until roughly age 10, after which there is a gradual decline so that by late adolescence half the synapses in the brain have been discarded, leaving about 500 trillion. This is in the non-clinical population.
>
> [Balbernie 2001, p. 240]

The Principal Methodologies of Parent-child Consultations

In order to organize the presentation of different modalities of treatment, I will utilize in part the outline proposed by Stern (1995) in his book on the "mother-hood constellation," that "special organization" of psychic life, adapted to the real situation of having a baby to care for. Stern differentiates therapeutic interventions according to the target of the intervention and the modality of entry into the parent-child system. In this presentation, I will limit myself to psychotherapeutic models aimed principally at the parents and their representations of the child or principally to the child's representations.

Interventions Aimed Principally at the Parents' Representations and the Parents' Representations as an Entry into the System

The first paper addressing parent-child interventions that came to my attention was by Bernard Cramer: "Interventions thérapeutiques brèves avec parents et enfantas" (1974).

Cramer, before definitively establishing himself in Geneva, had worked in the US with Margaret Mahler. In his early pioneering work, he had empha-sized the concept of *psychic mutuality*, which views the child as *a system open to* the influences of the early relationship, and the younger the child, the more this is true.

Consultations, according to Cramer, should start by gathering the anamnesis in an unstructured way that can promote free associations, during which the par-ents "reveal their investment in the child and the interplay of projections and introjections – identifications between parents and child" (1974, p. 94, translation by G. Atkinson).

In Cramer's opinion, brief therapies are especially indicated in cases in which the child's pathology appears basically connected to the pathogenic interference of parental phantasms who block the *demarrage:* the child's setting sail, as it were, in initiating processes of individuation.

From another part of the ocean, those phantasms have already acquired a name; they were the *phantasms of the children's room* – "ghosts in the nursery," according to the title of a wonderful article by Fraiberg et al. (1975). The opening words of this article have great impact:

> In every nursery there are ghosts. They are the visitors from the unremembered past of the parents: the uninvited guests at the christening. Under all favorable circumstances the unfriendly and unbidden spirits are banished from the nursery and return to their subterranean dwelling place. The baby makes his own imperative claim upon parental love and, in strict analogy with the fairy tales, the bonds of love protect the child and his parents against the intruders, the malevolent ghosts.
>
> [Fraiberg et al. 1975, p. 387]

Selma Fraiberg and her colleagues at the Mental Health Program of San Francisco (Lieberman et al. 2000) strongly advised giving considerable attention to the parent-child relationship, placing fantasies and maternal memories at the centre of their interventions. Lieberman and Pawl (1993; Lieberman et al. 2000), who studied Selma Fraiberg's work in San Francisco, encourage interventions that aim at "liberating the child from distortions and repressed affects that overwhelm them with parental conflict" or at "modifying internal representations that the parents have of themselves and of the child" (Fraiberg 1980, quoted in Stern 1995, p. 123).

The San Francisco group does not focus only on the parents' representations and their phantasms but also takes account of the child's contribution and proposes an "experience of corrective attachment." They introduced the child's presence into sessions, often held in the home, in this way causing the child to become the object of verbal interventions that encourage the parents' identification with the child's needs, at first obscured by the "phantasms" of their past. In this group's interventional philosophy, the child's presence determines a climate of emotional immediacy that is different from the tone of conversations with parents. (It must be said that their interventions were geared toward disadvantaged populations in San Francisco, and a positive pre-transference to the therapist and to the institution, which characterized the patients of their Swiss colleagues, could not always be counted on.)

Cramer's (1974) theorizations have recently been taken up again and reintroduced in Geneva, together with those of Francisco Palacio Espasa and Juan Manzano on therapeutic consultations, especially those dedicated to children of preschool age. The cultural background of colleagues in Geneva, firmly placed under the rubric of classical psychoanalysis, in addition to the already cited French paediatric and psychiatric psychoanalysts, refers to A. Freud, M. Klein, D. Winnicott, R. Spitz, J. Bowlby, M. Mahler, S. Fraiberg, and D. Meltzer.

They began from the assumption that early parent-child psychotherapeutic interventions were aimed at the relationship rather than the individual, and they had to be time-limited and could fulfil a preventative function in relation to the establishment of conflictual parent-child relationships before these relationships grew into more structured pathologies. The necessity for these interventions was born of the observation of clinical practice indicating that the major portion of consultations aimed at children under two years of age had an average duration of about six sessions, with a minimum of three and a maximum of twelve, while 75% of the consultations for children younger than age four ended after no more than ten sessions. A clinical sixth sense highlighted the potential preventative value of mother-child consultations; in favourable cases, the "symptomatic modifications are sometimes spectacular" (Palacio Espasa and Manzano 1982, p. 5). They are especially effective if the intervention is carried out at an early age, in depressed children, or with slowed psychomotor development following maternal depression.

Even if in more recent theorizations it has been stated that only in rare cases do early interventions represent a definitive solution to children's problems; these early interventions permit the parents to be much more open to their children's psychological and emotional needs (Knauber and Palacio Espasa 2002).

In fact, the mother requests a consultation for a symptom of the child's, not for her own symptom. Most often, postpartum psychic functioning is the area of intervention, where there is considerable maternal psychic mobilization, including an enormous capacity to establish connections and mobilize affects.

During this period, the rapidity of subjective, interactive, and symptomatic changes is astonishing, due to the elaboration of phantasms and of representations that the mother has had of the child. For the child present in treatment, an important role as a subject capable of bringing in his own contribution begins to be recognized. The child finds himself "liberated" from the attributions of instinctual or superego aspects split off from the mother or father or from the role of a parent's important figure toward whom mourning has not been adequately elaborated.

The Geneva group hypothesizes, in fact, that a large portion of early childhood psychopathology originates from the parents' "conflictual overburdening," which pours out onto the child through projections of the former onto the latter. Consultations can lessen their effect by helping to find less regressive solutions.

These colleagues have tried to identify situations that they see as indicating brief psychotherapeutic interventions; those in which such interventions are contraindicated; and those on the border. Their discrimination among these seems consistent whether or not a libidinal tie is present (however conflictual with the child), contrary to situations in which evacuative aspects prevail and the parents project onto the child something of which they would like to be liberated. In these latter cases, the suggestion of contact with evacuative elements projected onto the child pushes the parents to refuse any kind of therapy because they feel, unconsciously, that it would require pain and sorrow. In other words, there are identifications of a hysterical type, as opposed to projections that are more of a paranoid type.

Brief therapy, in the view of these theoreticians, is not indicated when there is a "negative pre-transference," often linked to serious maternal pathology (psychosis, seriously borderline structure, considerable psychosomatic disturbances, or intense depressions of a melancholy character). According to the Geneva group, situations are more sensitive to these interventions when "the child and especially his symptomatic configurations play a role in the mother's psychic economy, allowing her to again find and recover a lost object whose mourning is still conflictual" (Palacio Espasa and Manzano 1982, p. 9, translation by G. Atkinson).

The Role of the Parent: Acquisition of the Parental Role and Possible Areas of Weakness

When one finds oneself with parents who talk about their child's problems, one often has the impression of coping not with two generations but more generations, interwoven among themselves by a continuity of life experiences that lead to questions about the upbringing of the parents whom we are with now when they were little, as their child is now.

Acquiring the parental role is a synthesis of the process of development and maturation through which every individual, having gone through the different growth stages, then faces as he brings a child into the world – a child who, in addition to having his own potential and his own individual legacy, at the same time is already shaped by the representations of him that his parents have (D'Alberton and Roncarati 1992). In these fantasies pertaining to the new-born, always present are the parents whom the new parents had in their personal histories – and the way in which the relationship with them was experienced during various stages of development, especially early childhood and adolescence. Each of us, in fact, in our own childhood had to find a balance between realizing our desires and the requirements coming from those who have the task of educating us, and these are the conquests that at times cause us suffering and conflicts.

Even though there is a tendency to see childhood as a carefree age, we have been aware for some time that this phase of life is crisscrossed with tensions that are sometimes very strong, and in relation to these the child derives a great advantage from the presence of adults who allow him to sustain, give shape to, and transform life experiences.

The vicissitudes of love and aggressivity in psychosexual development involve as subjects the parental figures and the frustration of childhood desires. Placing limits on the child's behaviour is a part of their role that parents cannot evade; that role is certainly not to allow the child to do whatever he wants, nor should we avoid any opposition with those whom we are helping to grow.

Of course, the expectations and fantasies about the newly arrived child, if they are not too intense or distorted, promote the establishment of a connection with the child. Sometimes a period of revision and inner change opens up in which important moments of one's own childhood are relived; very old relationships can be enriched and transformed in light of the new relationship with the child – or, in contrast, they can repeat themselves in an identical manner.

Whether the representations that each person has of his own parents can remain in the background, on the one hand – following along with discretion and supporting the new relationship being created – or whether, on the other hand, these representations become an intrusive presence tied to the parents' complex narcissistic scenario (Manzano et al. 1999) or to the "narcissistic contract" that accompanies the child on his arrival into the world and inserts him into the transgenerational familial chain (Aulagnier 1975) – will depend on the result of the growth process and personal development, on the degree of integration and cohesion between various aspects of the self that are reached by the individual, and on a kind of mourning regarding the child's actual role.

When a child is born, there is often a kind of cross-identification, a sort of division between a part of the parent who takes on the role that his parents played in relation to him and a part of the parent that identifies with the child. Distortions in the parent-child relationship can arise when the presence of the child reactivates unresolved conflicts with one's own parents or causes intolerable or repressed aspects of one's personal history to reappear.

Of course, this is a question of degrees and intensity. All parents develop fantasies about the child; in the most favourable circumstances, the new parent identifies with the loving parent whom he himself had, and he sees in his son or daughter the loved child whom he felt himself to be. In this way, the parent renews the positive connection with his own parent.

Attributions to the son or daughter of aspects of the child whom the parents would have themselves wanted to be – and identifications with the parent whom they would have wanted to have – can lie at the foundation of some problems. These are people who have suffered due to aspects of their own parents that were too rigid or too permissive; they are the ones who tell us, "I don't want my children to suffer what I suffered." Difficulties may arise because underneath this positive availability toward the child, one can confuse the emotional reality of the parents' past with the child's current reality, running the risk of taking away from the child the possibility of expressing his own real needs.

Then there are other cases in which the parent says he does not want to be like his mother or his father and is tasked with not doing "what they would have done," as though a battle interrupted in adolescence were starting up again from new positions. These are often parents who want the child not to miss anything and suffer because the relationship with the child is not as good as they would like. In these cases, confusing one's own personal experience with that of the child keeps the parent from seeing that the child's problems are really the opposite of what the parent himself suffered – for example, that the child may need someone who helps him to set limits, to bear frustration, to delay the fulfilment of desires.

Interventions Aimed Primarily at the Child

One of the first people to emphasize the child's competence in interacting in the therapeutic consultation was Françoise Dolto (1971, 1985). A psychoanalyst akin to Lacan, Dolto tended to consider the child capable of intuiting his history and maintained that the child can grasp the meaning of the language of behaviours, gestures, and gazes. For Dolto, it was imperative to be authentic and sincere, and she recommended not lying to children because "one cannot lie to the unconscious; it always knows the truth," and the child perceives whether the truth is being told to him because "it is the truth that constructs him" (translation by G. Atkinson).

In a theoretical perspective in some ways different, one might locate Didier Houzel in the theoretical area of Melanie Klein and Wilfred Bion, with a direct link back to the methodology of observation developed by Esther Bick (1964). The formulation utilized by the "Under-Fives Consulting Service" of the Tavistock Clinic (Daws 1989; Miller 1992, 1994; Barrows 2003) was one in which – with a rather informal style and to the extent possible with brief appointments – up to five meetings of therapeutic consultations could be offered to parents who were worried about an aspect of their child's life. The parent-child consultations were distinguished from the system of traditional referrals at the Tavistock because the parents could self-refer to the service. Lisa Miller, referring to these experiences, maintains:

> One of the aspects of greatest satisfaction in working with small children is that, in a large number of cases, considerable change can be rapidly attained. In the intimacy of the early weeks, the early months and years, parents and children can be very open to change. It is probable that they look around themselves, unconsciously seeking a transferential object that can contain their anxieties and does not let them be overwhelmed.
> [1994, p. 155; translation by G. Atkinson]

In recent years, another object of attention in this field has been the work of Scandinavian colleagues, who try to focus on the competence of the child "as an active intentional agent" with the "capacity to contribute to the interaction and the process of the clinical situation" (Norman 2004, p. 1104). Their principal references are Bion, Klein, and Winnicott, with a link to more current literature through a collaboration with Allan Schore and his studies on the relationship between regulation of affect and the theory of attachment.

The psychoanalyst who most inspired this group was Johan Norman, who – in utilizing the concepts of containment, reverie, the oneiric waking dream, and transformation of alpha elements into beta elements – proposed a type of psychoanalysis of the new-born that does not reinvent a form of adult psychoanalysis or child psychoanalysis or a type of psychoanalytic psychotherapy. According to this author, the new-born demonstrates an innate capacity to locate himself in relation to the other, a trigger for being "contained" and for understanding nonverbal elements of language. For the first year to year-and-a-half of life, he is endowed with a unique plasticity that enables the possibility of modifying representations of self and other.

In the treatments that Norman puts forward, the analyst's communications are directed to the baby with the intention of reaching the parent, utilizing an analytic field that takes shape around the parent-baby relationship, the parent-analyst one, and the baby-analyst one, incorporating the topics of transference and countertransference implicit in all these situations.

In a paper published not long before his death, Norman described an analysis conducted at four sessions per week, over six weeks, with a six-month-old baby, Ossian. He was a baby who did not seem calm; he didn't sleep much and cried a lot, expressing suffering that the parents could neither understand nor ameliorate. Various doctors to whom the parents had turned told them that the baby was healthy – until they met with Norman, who took the situation in hand, explaining to the parents that he utilized a way of working that led him to address himself to the baby verbally in an attempt to establish a relationship with him in the parents' presence.

With reference to the Bionian theory of *learning from experience*, the interest that the baby demonstrated for Norman led him to maintain that baby and analyst were reciprocally connected by a linking knowledge (K). In the paper cited earlier, Norman described addressing himself to the infant, introducing himself and telling him that he could see he was attentive to him. He then explained that the mother had looked for something that worried her and probably worried him as well:

> Ossian, who looked at me attentively when I was talking with him, looked then at his mother, but rather soon he turned away from his mother and me and looked around the room. I followed what he was doing with my comments, quite simple descriptive comments, like ". . . and there is Mother, she is sitting there . . . you are looking around the room, you have never been here before. . . ." He began to relax and smiled at me and at his mother.
>
> [Norman 2004, pp. 1108]

What was described reminded me of a clinical fragment of my meeting with Giuseppe, a three-year-old who came to me together with his parents for symptoms that could lead to an area of the autistic spectrum. During the consultation, while Giuseppe explored the available toys alone, I told him that his mother and father had brought him to me because at times they saw him as absorbed and detached, and they wanted to understand, together with him, what was worrying him. When the child detached his gaze from the toys and looked at me, his mother, with a gesture of surprise, recounted that it was the first time she had seen her son interested in something. On the basis of this initial consultation, a therapy at three sessions per week was initiated.

Norman asserts that the changes that occur in such situations, in particular in the case described by him, can be attributed primarily to the fact that the fantasies and mental representations of the mother about the child were modified, and there was a reduction of her anxiety and utilization of intrusive projective identifications; defensively, a place was left for more functional, communicative projective identifications in a Bionian sense. The Scandinavian position is now led by Björn Salomonsson (2014), who has followed the path opened by Norman, applying it both in private practice and subsequently in health services.

Daniela Montelatici Prawitz (2014) helps us understand the characteristics of the work group of Stockholm colleagues. Initially, they saw parents and new-born babies in their private offices, with treatments of at least a few months at a high frequency. Then, even though their way of working continued to inspire treatments with multiple sessions per week, they began to operate in children's public health settings as well, in once-weekly meetings.

Public consultation clinics for early childhood and for pregnant women have a rich tradition in Sweden. Families are automatically connected with these services and then followed for years. The personnel in these clinics is composed of doctors and specialized nurses. In earlier years, there were psychologists connected to these clinics, but today the families who demonstrate problems of a psychological type are referred to child psychiatric centres. The nurses at public clinics are generally trained to catch psychic problems, especially depression.

In the Stockholm experience, families meet with a nurse to whom they are entrusted once a week during the first month, with a home visit as well. During the first four months, monthly contacts are planned, and during the rest of the early years, every two months. Afterward there are check-ups at a year and a half, at three, four, and five years. During these visits, the child's growth is checked, his weight is taken, and he is measured and given vaccinations and paediatric advice of various types. The majority of these families appreciate these opportunities and regularly attend the clinics. Groups of various types are also possible for the parents – for example, mothers alone or fathers alone, for baby massage, etc.

Based on the assumption that it is not easy for a parent to consult psychiatric services or to enter a psychoanalyst's office for a problem with their child, through a foundation's funding, this group succeeded in establishing a program in which ten psychoanalysts work one day a week in one of the clinics. In this way, each psychoanalyst has the possibility of seeing at least five families and providing supervision for the clinic's medical personnel.

Another meaningful project is Frances Salo's (2007) in Australia, following a line of thought that identifies the baby himself as the possible subject of an intervention with him. At Melbourne Royal Children's Hospital, an intervention is offered that employs "a twofold approach to understanding the infant's experience through interactive dialogue between therapist and infant, and sharing this understanding with the parents" (p. 961).

An Italian Experience: The Participatory Consultation

It is not possible to conclude this general survey of techniques of intervention with children and parents without referring to the work of Dina Vallino and her proposal of participatory consultation. This participatory consultation is aimed not only at the early childhood sector; at the same time, it is distinct from traditional therapy, but in some situations it also represents preparation for individual child therapy.

Participatory consultation was born as an extension of Esther Bick's method of infant observation and subsequent theoretical elaborations by Martha Harris and Donald Meltzer. It focuses on children – from the very young to pre-pubescence – and on their parents.

Fundamental for Vallino is the parents' participation in the session; child, mother, and father are seen as a small group.

With different points of view and meanings that require clarification, parents and children demonstrate that they are capable of following associative chains, and through fantasies and images, they address "phantasmatic familial life that connects the child and the parental couple in a cryptic way" (Vallino 2002, p. 327; translation by G. Atkinson).

In this way, the parents' participation is encouraged in the session's emotional atmosphere, making them participants in the observational modalities utilized by the therapist in working with children. This promotes an understanding of children's mental states, whose incomprehension often forms the basis of the suffering that has led the parents and their child to the consultation. The most typical consultation is usually conducted in five sessions or, at times, if necessary, in more sessions, becoming a prolonged participatory consultation.

After the meetings with the parent(s) and child, almost always there are meetings with the parents alone, in order to allow them to discuss with the therapist what has emerged in the conjoint sessions, utilizing as well the reading of a brief written document that the therapist offers on what happened in the preceding sessions. In this way, it becomes possible to treat, in the mind of the child, the core kernels of the "primary intrusive and alienating identifications" that alter his sense of identity. In an attitude of respectful waiting, along the lines of *negative capability* (Bion 1970), the analyst finds himself in the situation of letting go of "the imaginary stratifications of the symptom, in order to contact the symbolic and latent meaning in that phobia, in that inhibition" (Vallino 2002, p. 336; translation by G. Atkinson).

According to Vallino, the participatory consultation is not to be understood as family therapy or therapy for the parents but rather as a modality with which to activate a function of reverie that allows construction of new meanings of the child's behaviour; it is "a unique occasion for the child to speak about himself and for the parents to speak with him, with tools mediated by psychoanalytic thinking" (Vallino 2002, p. 325; translation by G. Atkinson).

Efficacy Research

While one has the impression of perceiving, at an empirical level, the intrinsic therapeutic potential of various forms of parent-child therapies, attempts to evaluate the efficacy of these with statistical methods have not been numerous. In this field as well, the Swiss have been leaders, starting from the early 1990s. Cramer's group (Cramer et al. 1990), in a research paper that has been cited over time (Stern 1995; Robert-Tissot et al. 1996), examined the effects of cycles of brief psychotherapeutic consultations (fewer than 10 sessions) on 75 mother-child dyads, evaluating at fixed intervals the results of interventions on the child's symptoms, behavioural interactions, and maternal representations. The results of these interventions have been compared to other interventions of an international nature according to McDonough's therapeutic model of interactive support (Stern 1995, p. 151). The results were good and long-lasting for both forms of therapy, without a great difference between the two types of treatment; both produced a symptomatic reduction, more harmonious mother-child interaction, and an increase in maternal self-esteem.

In a more recent contribution by the same group (Nanzer et al. 2012), the effect of a brief psychoanalytic therapy on maternal perinatal depression was evaluated, drawing on data from 129 pregnant women examined according to two scales: the Edinburgh Postnatal Depression Scale (EPDS) and the "Dépistage antenatale de la dépression postnatale." The 40 women who presented with significant depression values were offered four sessions of a form of therapy called "psychotherapy focused on parenthood" – two sessions before birth and two afterward. This group was then compared with a control group of 88 women without depressive symptoms. The EPDS was administered again at three months and six months after the birth, together with other scales evaluating parental functioning. The result was a notable drop in depression indicators, and none of the women in the treatment group met the threshold for depression at three or six months after the birth. In addition, all the dyads who were treated indicated well-adapted mother-baby relationships.

Additional data comes from research structured according to the Scandinavian model (Salomonsson and Sandell 2011; Salomonsson-Winberg et al. 2015), which compared two groups of mother-baby dyads in a randomized study. One group was offered mother-baby psychoanalytic treatment (MIP), and traditional treatment supportive of parenthood was offered to the other. Positive results were identified in maternal sensitivity, in improvement of depression experienced by the mother, and in evaluations by experts of the quality of the mother-baby relationship. The same babies were re-evaluated once they reached four and a half years of age with regard to the quality of attachment, socio-emotional development, and global functioning. The group that underwent treatment expressed better values in global functioning, and it emerged that there were more children who were doing well in the treated group and more children with problems in the untreated group. The conclusion was that a relatively brief mother-baby therapy seemed to help children function better three-and-a-half years after the initial therapy.

Similar results emerged from Cochrane's recent review of the efficacious effect of parent-child psychotherapy (PIP) on the mental health of both parent and child (Barlow et al. 2015), which examined the literature on this topic, targeting eight studies that included 846 randomized participants. This study identifies parent-child psychotherapy as a promising model for improving the security of attachment in children from at-risk families. Even though a statistically significant difference between untreated subjects and those treated with more traditional methods of assistance was not documented, the authors hope that more rigorous research will highlight the impact of parent-child therapy on important factors of mediation, such as parental mental health, reflective functioning, and parent-child interaction.

In clinical practice, on the other hand, one can experience the efficacy of this type of intervention each time that the connection between early infantile symptomatology and underlying parental representations is loosened, often leaving us amazed by the pathways that open up before a development that in the context of those dynamics seemed to be arrested.

References

Abraham, N. & Torok, M. (1978). *The Shell and the Kernel*, ed. & trans. N. T. Rand. Chicago, IL/London: University of Chicago Press, 1994.

Alexander, F. & French, T. M. (1946). *Psychoanalytic Therapy: Principles and Application*. Omaha, NE: University of Nebraska Press, 1980.

Aulagnier, P. (1975). *The Violence of Interpretation: From Pictogram to Statement*, trans. A. Sheridan. London: Institute of Psychoanalysis, 2001.

Balbernie, R. (2001). Circuits and circumstances: The biological consequences of early relationship experiences and how they shape later behaviour. *J. Child Psychother.*, 27:237–255.

Balint, M. (1957). *The Doctor, His Patient and the Illness*. London: Tavistock Publications.

Barlow, J., Bennett, C., Midgley, N., Larkin, S. & Wei, Y. (2015). Parent-infant psychotherapy for improving parental and infant mental health: A systematic review. *Campbell Systematic Reviews*, 11(6).

Barrows, P. (2003). Change in parent-infant psychotherapy. *J. Child Psychother.*, 29:283–300.

Bick, E. (1964). Notes on infant observation in psycho-analytic training. *Int. J. Psychoanal.*, 45:558–566.

Bion, W. (1970). *Attention and Interpretation. A Scientific Approach to Insight in Psycho-Analysis and Groups*. London: Tavistock Publications.

Bollas, C. (1987). *The Shadow of the Object: Psychoanalysis of the Unthought Known*. New York: Columbia University Press.

Bruno, G. & Norsa, D., eds. (2009). *La psicoterapia psicoanalitica madre-bambino: Prevenire e curare il disagio del bambino e del suo ambiente [Mother-Child Psychoanalytic Psychotherapy: Preventing and Treating the Discomfort of the Child and His Environment]*. Roma: Il Pensiero Scientifico.

Cena, L., Imbasciati, A. & Baldoni, F., eds. (2010). *La relazione genitore-bambino: Dalla psicoanalisi infantile a nuove propettive evoluzionistiche dell'attaccamento [The Parent-Child Relationship: From Infantile Psychoanalysis to New Evolutionary Perspectives on Attachment]*. Berlin: Springer Science & Business Media.

Cramer, B. (1974). Interventions thérapeutiques brèves avec parents et enfantas. *Psychiatrie de l'enfant*, 17:53–117.

Cramer, B. & Palacio Espasa, F. (1993). *Le psicoterapie madre bambino*. Milano: Masson, 1995.

Cramer, B., Robert-Tissot, C., Stern, D. N., Serpa-Rusconi, S., De Muralt, M., Besson, G., et al. (1990). Outcome evaluation in brief mother-infant psychotherapy: A preliminary report. *Infant Mental Health J.*, 11:278–300.

D'Alberton, F. (2016). Psicoanalisi in ospedale: prima adolescenza e disturbi somatici funzionali [Psychoanalysis in the hospital: Early adolescence and somatic functional disturbances]. *Rivista di Psicoanalisi*, 62:463–479.

D'Alberton, F. & Roncarati, A. (1992). Catene di dolore non pensato [Chains of unthought pain]. *Rivista di psicologia clinica*, 1(92).

Daws, D. (1989). *Nel corso della notte [In the Course of the Night]*. Napoli: Liguori, 1992.

de Ajuriaguerra, J. (1993). *Manuale di psichiatria del bambino [Manual of Child Psychiatry]*. Milano: Masson, 1979.

Dolto, F. (1971). *Psicoanalisi e pediatria [Psychoanalysis and Pediatrics]*. Milano: Bompiani, 1973.

———. (1985). *Le parole dei bambini e l'adulto sordo [The Words of Children and the Deaf Adult]*. Milano: Mondadori, 1988.

Eliot, L. (1999). *What's Going On in There? How the Brain and Mind Develop in the First Five Years of Life*. New York: Bantam Books.

Faimberg, H. (2005). *The Telescoping of the Generations: Listening to the Narcissistic Links Between Generations*. London: New Library of Psychoanalysis.

Ferenczi, S. (1932). *The Clinical Diary of Sándor Ferenczi*, ed. J. Dupont, trans. M. Balint & N. J. Jackson. Cambridge, MA: Harvard University Press, 1988.

Ferenczi, S. & Rank, O. (1923). *The Development of Psychoanalysis*. Classics in psychoanalysis monograph series, 1986.

Fonagy, P. & Target, M. (1997). Attachment and reflective function: Their role in self-organization. *Devel. Psychol.*, 9:679–700.

Fraiberg, S. (1980). *Clinical Studies in Infant Mental Health: The First Year of Life*. New York: Basic Books.

Fraiberg, S., Adelson, E. & Shapiro, V. (1975). Ghosts in the nursery: A psychoanalytic approach to the problems of impaired infant-mother relationships. *J. Am. Acad. Child Psychiatry*, 14:387–421.

Freud, S. (1892–1893). A case of successful treatment by hypnotism: With some remarks on the origin of hysterical symptoms through "counter-will". *S. E.*, 1.

———. (1893). Frau Emmy von N., case histories from *Studies on Hysteria. S. E.*, 2.

———. (1923). Two encyclopaedia articles. *S. E.*, 18.

Golse, B. (2006). *L'étre bébé*. Paris: Presses Universitaires de France.

Homer (c. 762 BC). *The Iliad*, trans. A. T. Murray. Cambridge, MA/London: Harvard University Press/William Heinemann, 1924. www.perseus.tufts.edu/hopper/text?doc=Perseus%3Atext%3A1999.01.0134%3Abook%3D1%3Acard%3D345

Houzel, D. (2010). *L'Eredità psichica [Psychic Heredity]*. Roma: Armando, 2011.

Knauber, D. & Palacio Espasa, F. (2002). Interventions précoces parents-enfants: Avantages et limites. *La psychiatrie de l'enfant*, 45(1):103–132.

Kreisler, L. (1981). *Clinica psicosomatica del bambino [Clinical Psychosomatics in the Child]*. Milano: Raffaello Cortina, 1986.

Kreisler, L., Fain, M., Soulé, M. & Lebovici, S. (1974). *L'enfant et son corps: études sur la clinique psychosomatique du jeune âge*. Paris: Presses universitaires de France.

Lebovici, S., Diatkine, R. & Soulé, M. (1985). *Traité de psychiatrie de l'enfant et de l'adolescent, II*. Paris: Presses universitaires de France.

Lieberman, A. F. & Pawl, J. H. (1993). Infant-parent psychotherapy. In *Handbook of Infant Mental Health*, ed. C. H. Zeanah. New York: Guilford, 2005, pp. 427–442.

Lieberman, A. F., Silverman, R. & Pawl, J. H. (2000). Infant-parent psychotherapy: Core concepts and current approaches. In *Handbook of Infant Mental Health*, ed. C. H. Zeanah. New York: Guilford, 2005, pp. 472–484.

Magnini, L. & Sala, A. (2013). Un modello di consultazione familiare per l'infanzia [A model of family consultation for childhood]. In *Psicoterapia psicoanalitica dell'età evolutivo, Clinica e Formazione [Psychoanalytic Psychotherapy during the Developmental Age: Clinical Work and Training]*, ed. A. Sala & E. Albertini. Milano: Mimesis.

Mahler, M., Pine, F. & Bergman, A. (1975). *The Psychological Birth of the Human Infant: Symbiosis and Individuation*. London: Routledge.

Manzano, J., Espasa, F. P. & Zilkha, N. (1999). The narcissistic scenarios of parenthood. *Int. J. Psychoanal.*, 80:465–476.

Migone, P. (2004). Le differenze tra psicoanalisi e psicoterapia breve psicoanalitica [The differences between psychoanalysis and brief psychoanalytic psychotherapy]. In *Terapia psicoanalitica [Psychoanalytic Therapy]*. Milano: FrancoAngeli.

Miller, L. (1992). The relation of infant observation to clinical practice in an under five counselling centre service. *J. Child Psychother.*, 18:19–32.

———. (1994). Il "servizio 0–5." In *Un buon incontro: La valutazione secondo il modello Tavistock [A Good Meeting: Evaluation According to the Tavistock Model]*, ed. A. Alvarez & B. Copley. Roma: Astrolabio.

Missonier, S. (2003). *La consultazione terapeutica perinatale [Therapeutic Perinatal Consultation]*. Milano: Raffaello Cortina, 2005.

Montelatici Prawitz, D. (2014). La consultazione protratta a futuri genitori e a genitori e figli in tenera età [Long-term consultation to future parents and to parents and children of a young age]. Paper given at Bologna Psychoanalytic Center, October 3. www.spiweb.it/eventi/3-ottobre-2014-cpb-giornata-sulla-consultazione-protratta-a-futuri-genitori-e-a-genitori-e-figli-in-tenera-eta/.

Moro, A. M. (1994). *Genitori in esilio [Parents in Exile]*. Milano: Raffaello Cortina, 2002.

Nanzer, N., Rossignol, A. S., Righetti-Veltema, M., Knauer, D., Manzano, J., Espasa, F. P. (2012). Effects of a brief psychoanalytic intervention for perinatal depression. *Archives of Women's Mental Health*, 15:259–268.

Norman, J. (2004). Transformations of early infantile experiences: A 6-month-old in psychoanalysis. *Int. J. Psychoanal.*, 85:1103–1122.

Palacio Espasa, F. & Manzano, J. (1982). La consultation thérapeutique des très jeunes enfants et leur mère [Therapeutic consultations with babies and their mothers]. *La Psychiatrie de l'Enfant*, 25:5–25.

Pellizzari, G. (2009). *La seconda nascita. Fenomenologia dell'adolescenza [Second Birth: The Phenomenology of Adolescence]*. Milano: FrancoAngeli.

Robert Tissot, C., Cramer, B., Stern, D. N., Serpa, S. R., Bachmann, J. P., Palacio Espasa, F., et al. (1996). Outcome evaluation in brief mother infant psychotherapies: Report on 75 cases. *Infant Mental Health J.*, 17:97–114.

Salo, F. T. (2007). Recognizing the infant as subject in infant-parent psychotherapy. *Int. J. Psychoanal.*, 88:961–979.

Salomonsson, B. (2014). *Psychoanalytic Therapy with Infants and Their Parents: Practice, Theory, and Results*. London/New York: Routledge.

Salomonsson, B. & Sandell, R. (2011). A randomized controlled trial of mother-infant psychoanalytic treatment: I. Outcomes on self-report questionnaires and external ratings. *Infant Mental Health J.*, 32:207–231.

Salomonsson-Winberg, M. W., Sorjonen, K. & Salomonsson, B. (2015). A long-term follow-up of a randomized controlled trial of mother-infant psychoanalytic treatment: Outcomes on the children. *Infant Mental Health J.*, 36:12–29.

Soubieux, M. J. & Soulé, M. (2005). *La psichiatria fetale [Fetal Psychiatry]*. Milano: FrancoAngeli, 2007.

Stern, D. N. (1995). *The Motherhood Constellation: A Unified View of Parent-Infant Psychotherapy*. London/New York: Routledge, 1998.

Vallino, D. (2002). Percorsi teorico-clinici sul trauma [Theoretical-clinical journeys on trauma]. *Rivista di Psicoanalisi*, 48:5–22.

Winnicott, D. W. (1965). Utility of the therapeutic consultation. In *Psychoanalytic Explorations*, ed. C. Winnicott, R. Shepherd & M. Davis. Abingdon, UK/New York: Routledge, 2018.

———. (1971). Convulsions, fits. In *The Collected Works of D. W. Winnicott, Vol. 10: Therapeutic Consultations in Child Psychiatry*, ed. L. Caldwell & H. T. Robinson. New York: Oxford University Press, 2017.

Chapter 8

Parent-child Consultations
Addiction to Liquids

Potomania, addiction to liquids – or psychogenic *polidypsia*, abnormal thirst – is a disturbance of ingesting liquids, which can present in early childhood and which leads an individual to consume great quantities in a way that can't be explained by medical causes. In childhood, this condition is more frequently seen in the hospital, because children are brought there to rule out the presence of organic conditions such as diabetes mellitus or diabetes insipidus, which can be expressed with similar symptomatology.

In what follows, two cases of small children will be presented – children treated with different modalities of parent-child consultation, almost to emphasize the versatility of that treatment method that lends itself to coping with every situation in the most appropriate way in relation to the exigencies and therapeutic possibilities.

Elton: A Unique Encounter

Elton had been hospitalized because at age two, he would drink from five to seven litres of water a day, of which two were consumed at night. A series of clinical tests and procedures had ruled out the presence of diabetes, whether of the mellitus type or insipidus, and his caregivers sent him to our clinical service because they hypothesized the presence of a psychogenic potomania.

Elton presented to the consultation with his parents. He was a thin child, alert, very intelligent, with language that was slightly below the norm for his age. He presented not only with the problem of excessive drinking, but also with prolonged constipation treated with medications to soften his bowel movements, which were eliminated only after administration of a daily enema. At first sight, then, there was a sleep problem and an elimination problem.

The parents seemed willing to consider the influence of emotional factors because they had noticed that Elton's drinking requirement was lessened when he was with his grandparents.

In the course of our meeting, while the child organized his toys, the parents described an objectively complicated living-relational situation. They came from two different areas of Italy; they had married in the city where the mother lived

DOI: 10.4324/9781003252238-9

with her parents, and where Elton had been born and lived for his first year with his mother and maternal grandparents. The father had been intermittently present because he worked in a city in central Italy, where he was trying to set up a living situation such that the new nuclear family could eventually move there. The relational nucleus in which the little boy had lived during his first year of life had been that of the mother's family, characterized by the presence of constantly available adults; this environment suddenly went missing once the parents were finally able to reunite in the city in which they had chosen to live.

This change in the physical and relational environment had not been easy, and according to the father's report, a struggle had begun over what he had to do to "make himself acceptable" to a son whom he hardly knew.

Elton had been born at the forty-second week of his mother's pregnancy and had been breastfed for a little more than a month; the mother's milk seemed not to satisfy him, and the paediatrician advised first a mixture and later a substitution of artificial milk. Since that time, there had been constipation problems, aggravated by the fact that, although he had eaten a varied diet while younger, over time he had become more selective and tended to reject fruits and vegetables.

An identification appeared to be constant over the course of the meeting, in that the mother saw herself as having had the same problems as her son: "I, too, was slender, I didn't eat much, and I was very rebellious."

Elton had never cared for a pacifier, and when he was nervous or angry, his demand for water increased; his parents came to see this as "a defense against momentary suffering."

The little boy would go to sleep with his cheek leaning against that of his mother, and he would awaken five or six times per night – something that did not bother his mother much, however, because she could rest during the day since she didn't work outside the home. The father, who was establishing his place within the couple in relation to the child, slept in a separate room in order to be able to rest, leaving the child "attached" to his mother. The mother did not seem overly resentful of the continual awakenings – not only because she could rest during the day, but also because she was buoyed by a strong identification with her own mother, in addition to identifying with her child: "I didn't sleep very much as a small child, and I see myself in Elton."

In this context, the father struggled to create a space for himself; the paternal figure appeared to be weakened, while the child's libidinal connection with his mother remained absolutely dominant. In the course of our meeting, a tendency also emerged to find justifications for various behaviours of Elton's. In the end, even his language delay seemed to characterize a child who had not experienced great frustrations of his need to make himself understood, immersed as he was in a relational environment of adults who were completely at his disposal, wanting only to fulfil his every desire.

If during child development, the experience of the absence of the primary object is necessary in order for symbolization and thinking to develop, in the case of Elton, sensations tied to the passage of liquids through the gastroesophageal tract – and the consequent sensation of fullness of the stomach – seemed to negate this at a concrete level. A shared system of negation probably led the family to undervalue the consequences for the child of the sudden change in his relational environment, which had been dealt with by a hypercompensation of maternal caregiving.

It would seem that the function of frustration and absence was missing in Elton's case – the function that pushes children to develop thinking and ego functions, such as language and transitionality (Winnicott 1953). The transitional function defines the intermediate area between internal reality and external reality, between the *purely subjective* and objectivity, and it helps the child tolerate the experience of aloneness by turning to a transitional object, such as Linus's blanket, which releases him from the necessity of the presence of and contact with the maternal body.

Due to the considerable distance that the family had to travel to this meeting, there were no further meetings. The parents were advised to contact a colleague in their area in order to bolster the newly formed nuclear family and to reinforce the parental couple who could help Elton cope with subsequent developmental stages with greater competence.

Jenny: An Enduring Treatment over the Years

In contrast, prolonged parent-child treatment was utilized in the case of Jenny. A little before summer vacation some years ago, at two-and-a-half years of age, Jenny had been hospitalized for suspected insipid diabetes – from the time that she started to drink a great deal of water, even at night, awakening frequently and asking for a drink. In her case, too, clinical examinations seemed to exclude an organic component, and the doctors advised the mother to contact me.

The mother did this somewhat against her will; on the phone, a certain reluctance was perceptible in setting an appointment. Then, with an eye toward the imminence of summer vacation, given that there was no rush, we agreed that we could observe how the situation unfolded, and if there was still a need, the mother would contact me after their return from vacation.

The First Meeting

In actuality, although she readily admitted to having tried not to do it, the mother called me at the beginning of September because she felt that she needed help for Jenny, her only child. When I met with the parents, they first talked to me about breathing problems that Jenny had had soon after her birth, which had occurred by Cesarean section some weeks before term due to a health problem of the mother's. Jenny had been a wanted child – "even too much so," according to her parents – leaving it to be intuited how much importance they attached to their daughter's birth, which the mother's health seemed not to want to permit. They described Jenny during the first year and a half of her life as a calm child who "ate and slept," who had attended day care "without problems," starting early due to the necessity for the mother to return to a very busy job. According to the parents, it seemed that Jenny barely registered the detachment from them; that she got along well with other children; and that all went well until 18 months of age, when a lung problem took her to the hospital. About the hospitalization, the parents remembered their daughter's being very upset, her high fever, the painful injections, and especially the beginning of a frequent demand for liquids, which did not abate and which worried them, particularly at night. From that point onward, Jenny would wake up from two to eight times a night and could not go back to sleep unless each time she was given a drink of water, which she gulped down in one breath.

In the parents' account, there had been a moment of silence that it seemed important to me to respect; as often happens in consultations, the experience of emptiness is fundamental to allow space for the emergence of thoughts that have not yet been thought. On these occasions, something only faintly there can often be expressed, part of the journey that a thought must sometimes undergo in order to be thought, awaiting meanings for which it is the carrier to be capable of taking shape.

After a while, the father invited the mother to speak of how she, too, had begun to drink a great deal during her pregnancy. The mother acquiesced and added that she had had to have at her side at least a bottle of water; otherwise, "I felt bad and, five minutes after I drank, I was thirsty again." That intense need to drink had ended on the day when she gave birth, and since then her level of thirst had returned to normal. The mother's story continued with the description of her clinical history of an organic pathology that had led her to undergo several surgeries, and for which she still had to adhere to close monitoring.

In addition, according to Jenny's parents, the emotional climate in the family affected the child's condition because, during the summer period when they were calmer she drank less, and once they resumed work, the management of the home and everyone's daily activities became more chaotic and increased Jenny's need to drink – something that, furthermore, rarely happened while she was in day care.

The mother further contributed by describing the child's many areas of competence. From four months of age, Jenny had no longer used a diaper during the day, while continuing to wear one at night in order not to be changed too many times.

The second of the siblings in her family, the mother had a brother five years older than herself. After a long period of poor health and lengthy hospitalizations, the mother, at age one-and-a-half – during a hospital stay for bronchitis – was diagnosed with significant pathology. This discovery had given rise to a series of interventions and further hospitalizations that lasted for years.

At this point I intervened, saying:

> I wonder what you must have felt when Jenny was brought to the hospital at the same age that you were when you were hospitalized, when your organic problem was diagnosed? I can imagine a great fear that what had happened to you could also happen to your daughter.

The mother seemed surprised by my intervention, remaining engrossed and thoughtful, and she resumed her account by confiding her impression that her health conditions had played a role in the deterioration of her relationship with her own parents, who in the course of her childhood had separated.

In the meeting, the mother ended up admitting that she felt very tired and was struggling to maintain the rhythm of her work life, not sleeping well at night. She confessed that at times "some bad thoughts" took hold of her, alluding to an intense irritation toward her daughter that led her to distance herself from her out of a fear of doing something rash. At those times she called her husband, who took account of the situation and tried to take care of the child, even though she would have preferred her mother.

The father listened to the mother's account – agreeing from time to time – and then talked about what a sensitive child Jenny was, capable of becoming very moved, as happened when she saw scenes of separation on television – for example, when Heidi was separated from her grandfather, or when Masha thought that as a grown-up she would have to be separated from Orso.

The Second Meeting

After this meeting, we agreed to embark on a series of consultations, with a session every two weeks – one with the parents together with Jenny and one with only the parents.

At the next session, Mom, Dad, and Jenny arrived on time. The parents immediately said that they were almost afraid to say that for several nights, things had gone better. Two nights earlier, Jenny had awakened only one time, and for them this was an unusual thing that made them happy. The mother then told of having spoken to their daughter and explained that she must try to sleep because if the mom didn't sleep well, she wouldn't be able to play with her much. With an air of amazement, they reported that the previous night, Jenny awoke only two times; on the first occasion, they had given her a drink, and on the second they managed to get her to go back to sleep without one.

Jenny presented as a sweet child, attentive, substantially secure, lively, and with excellent language skills. The first toys that she played with were a big baby doll with a baby bottle, to whom she gave a drink, and a big dinosaur with a wide-open mouth, who in the course of their play "will eat Mom." Then she explored other toys meticulously and with precision. Her parents watched, participating in her play – the mother more actively and the father with more discretion.

At the end of the session, in the hallway, the mother came close to me to tell me something that she had not said the previous time: "Jenny was born at 9:00 in the morning, and because of respiratory problems, I could see her only after a day and a half."

The meeting had ended and there was no time to deepen our discussion, but the idea that a fear of the child's death might still be alive and present had for some time hovered in my thoughts and had led me to think that Jenny's hospital stay might have represented a source of intense worry for the mother – who, during a similar hospitalization for a medical work-up, had experienced the discovery of her own health problem. The need to drink seemed to be induced more by something that had passed through the mother's mind than by an autonomous action of the child's. As often happens, important issues were presented at the moment of leaving, deposited there once the person is convinced that she can have faith in the other person and can trust him temporarily with emotional burdens that are difficult to carry.

The Third Meeting

At the next meeting, the parents arrived more calm; things were continuing to go well, and at most Jenny awakened once or twice per night. For example, the previous night she had not woken up at all, and the parents had awakened suddenly in the morning, asking themselves with surprise if something could have happened.

I then reminded the mother of what she had told me on leaving the office the previous time – about her worry over not having been able to see the child for a day and a half after her birth. She confirmed this and related that, after the Cesarean section, she had not been capable of moving to go and see her child. Even though she had been connected to many medical devices, she had insisted very strongly, to the point that she had been brought to see her daughter first in an incubator and then in intensive care, where she had subsequently been placed for respiratory problems. While this emergence of memories emotionally involved the father as well, the little girl had begun to take out toys and organize them. She had taken a doll and begun to feed her with a bottle, and subsequently placed some objects inside the big, wide-open jaws of threatening dinosaurs, a toy that she had put into a corner. It was as though in the game she had shown the need to take care of a little girl with whom she identified, satisfying her oral needs, and keeping at bay aggressive and angry oral impulses. These mechanisms did not escape the mother, who recounted that Jenny used to use punching and kicking to express her rage, while now she used words. This happened, for example, one time when the mother was talking on her cell phone, and Jenny, instead of getting angry, told her mother that she did not want her to be on the phone when she was with her – rejecting a mom who was physically close but emotionally distant, engaged in other things.

Two Sessions Later

At our fifth meeting, the situation was no longer as calm. For some nights, the parents had had little sleep because the child woke up again many times, asking for water, and they described situations that greatly annoyed the mother. Resorting to enormous rationalization, the mother told of "having agreed" with Jenny that she would put a nice big bottle – "an adult's bottle," a kind of flask – onto the bedside table, as well as a bigger night light, so that if the little girl woke up to drink, she could do so on her own. Here the symptom came to be confused with what underlay it, exchanging an emotional request with a request for liquids and thinking that a negotiation about liquids would have helped the child to pull herself out of it alone. Predictably, the method didn't work, and reciprocal irritations and expressions of anger sprang forth. In the face of this discomfort of the mother's, I, too, was a little surprised by the sudden breakdown of being in contact with the child's demands, and while I reflected on her apparently resigned mortification, the father intervened to say that, in his view, the child probably wanted her mother, not water. While we thought about this together, Jenny played near her mother, to whom she had entrusted a little doll, carefully giving her drinks from a bottle and admonishing her not to drink too quickly so as not to make herself vomit. Then the little girl asked for a drink herself and took one; as Jenny had done with her baby doll, her mother got up to give her some water and asked her to drink only a little and not all at once. Over the course of the meeting, the parents continued to remark on the fact that it was difficult that here there was a need for liquids, given that during the day, Jenny by now usually didn't ask to drink any more.

The child listened to what was said, now and then trying to attract our attention with direct and pertinent comments that aroused at the same time admiration and the feeling that she, too, was trying to shift the conversation onto the level of rationalization.

When the mother asked if the fact that she herself had drunk a lot during her pregnancy could have influenced her daughter's current behaviour – here, too, shifting to the physical level something that would have had more connection to the level of fantasy, I found myself asking her whether she remembered any thoughts related to those episodes. After some initial hesitation, the mother said that during that period, there had been great uncertainty about whether she would have to give birth by Cesarean section or in the natural way, "like other women." The specialists who had treated her since childhood maintained that her conditions would allow her to have natural childbirth, while the endocrinologists and gynaecologists were more disposed toward the alternative. Then, when the hypothesis cropped up of a previously unknown gestational diabetes, the idea of natural childbirth was excluded, then again proposed, then once more excluded until a very short time before the birth. This was a period in which the mother stopped working while she underwent a panoply of exhausting visits, almost daily, with various specialists, in search of someone who would take responsibility for authorizing a natural birth. The father lobbied for a Cesarean, worried about his wife's conditions and about the baby; in the end, according to him, "fortunately" the birth had been by Cesarean, given that at birth an episode of respiratory stress had occurred. The immediate period after the birth had been very problematic, with dissociative moments in which the mother, to give me an idea of it, said that she "saw herself from outside." She wanted to get out of bed, to go to her daughter, and her husband ended up pinning her down in order to prevent her from getting up while she was still attached to monitors and infusion equipment.

While we talked about these things, Jenny participated in the conversation, turning to her father almost as though to ask his help – bringing him monsters, ferocious animals that she hadn't used with her mother, almost asking him to take charge of her rage, which she feared was destructive. She also consigned to him a big dinosaur that she stated was good, even though he had a big mouth.

I reconnected with what the mother had said earlier when she tried to express the thought that maybe these painful memories could lead her to interpret the child's demands in terms of liquids, instead of being about maternal presence and reassurance, or that her memories could have impaired her understanding of the little girl's discomfort in missing her. The mother remembered that, essentially, taking a drink had always been a way for her to calm herself, even when she was little; in situations of difficulty, she often asked for something to drink – to such a degree that her grandparents, when she went to see them, always had a glass of water ready for her. The mother also remembered that they had told her that, in her maternal lineage, drinking a lot of water had been characteristic of the women of earlier generations, with the exception of her own mother. This raised questions about a possible genetic incidence of a low-grade form of diabetes insipidus, and about the possibility of a telescoping of the generations (Faimberg 2006) – that is, a representation in the course of therapy of unrepresentable psychic elements, experiences, or emotions that had belonged to previous generations.

However, I concentrated on what was happening in the consultation, and thinking of the mother's need to drink during her pregnancy, I asked myself whether refilling her mouth and stomach with water could be similar to what Jenny was doing – putting something into the dinosaur's mouth to neutralize some of the anxieties connected to aggression.

The session was ending when the mother reminded me that today's meeting was the next to the last of our agreed-upon sequence. She asked me whether the last meeting, which we had arranged to hold with the child as well because it fell on a day when we thought the schools would be closed, could instead be for the two of us only, given that the schools would be open after all. I agreed and took the opportunity to communicate the possibility of continuing our meetings, which in my mind was a given. The mother's surprised "*But is that OK?*" made me think that, in effect, for her it wasn't a given and that the difficulties of the recent period could be connected to her feeling that the interruption of our meetings would involve a new and painful separation, this time from me. In some manner, I too had left a bottle "for adults" on the table, from which she would have to quench her thirst autonomously. It had seemed greatly reassuring, however, to be able to count on the continuity of our relationship in coping with the anxieties that did not allow her to differentiate her own difficulties from those of her child.

The next meeting, which was held after a vacation break – with the parents only – effectively confirmed the correctness of the hypothesis about a feeling of abandonment on the mother's part. During the vacation period, things had gone particularly well: the emotional climate in general had been decidedly good,

Jenny woke up less frequently, and it happened that, through a gradually more developed language, the little girl managed to communicate by translating into emotional terms what had earlier been expressed as a concrete need for water.

Having begun with a description of how affectionate the child was – the child who with adult language and at times with a kind of role reversal said to her mother, "You're my love, you're my life, how lucky I am to have a family like this one" – we had reached the point of talking about how the child's birth represented for the mother a kind of precious miracle, but one that was constantly threatened by toxic experiences from her own clinical and personal history. She then said that our meetings had been important to her, having helped her orient herself in relation to something that didn't seem to make sense, and they helped her become able to come up with answers.

To have connected her own experience of hospital contact with her daughter's experience had been both moving and traumatic for the mother. She said:

> When I realized it after we had talked about it here, I cried for an entire day, and when I talked to my mother about it, she pointed out some things of which I hadn't been fully aware. My mom told me that something happened in the course of Jenny's hospitalization – that when I took her to get an x-ray, I went into the hall of the radiology department, which I knew very well because it was the same place where I had gone as a child. At that time, parents couldn't stay with their children, and I had cried desperately; my mother was forced to stay just outside the door. And so when I took my daughter there, I felt blocked and couldn't manage to move forward – to the point that my mother asked me what I was doing and told me to hurry up. I had been buried in a kind of confusion; I had a sort of déjà vu, as though I had essentially already lived through the situation.

Then the mother talked to me about an intense fear that Jenny might have the same physical problems that she herself had and her fear that she wasn't sufficiently capable of supporting her, as her own mother had been. The meeting ended with our agreeing to another series of meetings, alternating those that included the child and the parents with those where only the parents were present, for six subsequent months.

At one of those sessions, the mother said how much the child had wanted to come along and how she often talked about the toys at the sessions. In fact, as soon as she arrived, Jenny had taken out a big baby doll, the one with the bottle, and had given it to her mom. Then the child took out another one, and a third one she gave to her father. It was necessary to feed these little children and to take care of them, changing their diapers. The theme of these dolls would end up being the red thread of almost all our subsequent meetings, making an appearance in both prologue and conclusion.

While the little girl continued looking for toys in the box, the parents said that her sleeping was variable during different periods; now she was in a good period, though some months earlier there had been a worsening in which she again slept very little.

In the course of the session, Jenny moved around a lot, making strange movements with her body and repeating an unintelligible word, which we would come to discover was the title of a theatrical play she had seen. The play was about two brothers who met a scary ghost and saved themselves by doing comical dances while repeating the word.

In talking about the ghost, Jenny repeated emphatically, "the ghost is a man" – almost as though she wanted me to understand that the ghost had assumed a body and was personified in her internal world, having moved from being a bundle of persecutory sensations to becoming a character in her internal world.

At a certain point, the father asked her to give him a rubber puppet of a man, which he said that he liked a lot. I imagined this as a way of introducing his role as a man/father, separating himself from the mom/dad that had been entrusted to him at the beginning, when he too had been asked to hold a doll. It seemed to me a way to introduce sexual and generational differentiation – causing the appearance, in the relationship between mother and child, of the presence of a third who could help her distinguish herself. In order to do this, the child looked for a play figure in the drawer to which she had relegated, without naming them, "the bad ones." These were the dinosaurs that she had used in games during the first sessions in order to locate oral aggression in a specific part of our relational field. Once the dinosaurs were deposited there, she tended to avoid "taking them out a lot" subsequently, placing them near her father and putting things into their mouths, almost to keep them from closing their jaws and biting something. While she looked for the puppet, I marvelled at the new progress in our journey toward symbolization, when she could say, "I'm afraid of dinosaurs." I wondered if the dinosaur represented her aggressive oral impulses or perhaps those of her mother, from whom she did not feel differentiated.

Now Jenny's fears could be expressed and shared – just as when she woke up at night, she could say she was afraid instead of asking for something to drink. When she went to bed, she now asked to sleep with a light on and to have the curtains raised a little so that the room would not be in total darkness. Sometimes she asked to have taken away the clothes that she said reminded her of the ghost's clothes; through psychic mechanisms, she managed to keep at bay fears that were now, at least in part, mentally and verbally representable.

That session ended with Jenny playing with – and again affectionately taking care of – the baby dolls. One doll was hers, while another went to her mother and one to her father. She caressed the dolls and in turn they caressed her. She thus seemed to have internalized the technique of maternal care that had been liberated from the "ghosts in the nursery," as described by Selma Fraiberg and her colleagues (1975).

After a meeting that didn't take place because the little girl had a fever, at the next meeting, which had been arranged for the parents only, the mother came alone because the father was tied up at work. She told me that things had not been going well at home. After a rather long period of calm sleep, for the previous two weeks, Jenny had again been waking up at night, sometimes asking her mother for cuddles and sometimes for water. The mother appeared exasperated by these continual awakenings, which provoked resentment and anger toward her daughter – feelings that she was often unable to keep in check. This was even more the case because at those moments, Jenny violently refused her father's presence, kicking and screaming, whereas the father wanted to intervene so that the mother would not have to get out of bed.

As a consequence of the frequent awakenings, Jenny's bowel control had also gotten worse, while during the day "she seemed another child"; she was sociable and gladly went to day care, where she didn't ask for water – not even during the afternoon snack time.

When the mother tried to speak with her again about what was happening during the night, the little girl seemed to take great responsibility onto herself, promising that she would not call her mother or agreeing to strategies that unfailingly didn't work – such as that of buying a new bottle, an "adult" one, to put on the nightstand next to her bed. These "rational" ideas would dissolve when at night something very similar to an anxiety attack led her to forget everything and ask for her mother's presence/water.

For her part, the mother had noticed that: "There are nights when I am transformed and get very angry. I say things that I don't mean. Anger, sleepiness, tiredness."

In this regard, the mother seemed to be aware that for herself, too – not just for her daughter – a deep feeling, not listened to, could arise from the unconscious and shatter rational ideas into fragments.

I tried to propose a connection between the child's anxieties and the mother's – such as when, during the mother's pregnancy, she had wanted to drink a lot and became angry if someone didn't give her water. This had come up with her brother, who had tried to suggest that she drink less. The mother thus confirmed that, following along in the family tradition, as a youngster she too had habitually drunk a great deal.

Drinking made her feel good. Before she began to study, she would always drink a glass of water; and, before it was in vogue, in college she used a capacious bag to carry a one-and-a-half-litre bottle.

When, following my associations to Winnicott's (1953) transitional function, I found myself asking the mother whether Jenny had something that she wanted to keep nearby and that consoled her when she was in bed, she answered in the negative. But some content around these themes was circulating between us because immediately afterward, she said that after 30 years, she had found herself "restoring Ciccino to service" – speaking of a little bear, a transitional object she had used when she was little and that she still kept. She had told Jenny that the rather worn-out little bear had been the mother's and had been a companion to her when, as a child, it was time for her to go to sleep.

Almost to emphasize her reclaiming of split elements in her personal history, elements that had ended up with the child, the mother continued by saying:

> I, too, kept my parents from sleeping for a long time. I wanted to be awake – I didn't want to lie down, maybe partly because of my physical problems, due to which I felt I was suffocating when I lay down. My brother remembers that I would often find myself in my parents' room, where I would spend the night seated on the bed while they slept. I remember that the first time I slept all night was with my maternal grandparents, while Jenny, with her grandparents, is the same as she is at home. Perhaps only with her aunt, who has a very firm personality, does she sleep better. It should be said that her grandparents, both maternal and paternal, are happy to have her and let her do whatever she wants.

In this account, the mother's evocation of the nocturnal episode of her childhood led me to imagine that a more developed mother-child relationship had been threatened when an increase in anxious tension again sparked an identification with the deprived child whom the mother had felt herself to be in relation to a mom who was not very capable of being close to her. When such identifications predominated under stress, her maternal skills slipped and made her incapable of supporting her daughter. Mother and daughter appeared to be without defences when oral aggressive fantasies, imbued with death anxiety, burst into the relationship. Now in the session, the mother managed to achieve contact, speaking of the fear of wolves that her daughter often expressed in her play or through dinosaurs, which were always present in the background of our meetings.

At the end of this session, I asked myself whether the two previous negative weeks described by the mother might be connected to what was happening in the relationship between us, going back to the time that the rhythm of our sessions slowed due to my illness. That might convey an idea of how important the relationship with me had become for the mother – as though I were felt to be a nourishing bottle at her disposal. Such transferential elements probably leaned on previous relationships with doctors at my institution; over the course of her entire life, they had represented not only important reference points for her physical survival, but at times, they had also given her bad news and recommended painful interventions and treatments. Therefore, I imagined that when the relationship with me came to be seen as precarious, the split elements could not find containment and went back to ending up with the child.

Given the lack of continuous and satisfying nourishment, the relationship with Jenny was inundated by buried remnants, unrepresented inscriptions, and split traces of early traumas that no longer held together impulses of love and of hatred, causing a prevalence of toxic aggressive aspects over libidinal ones. The child thus returned to earlier identifications with a mother who, when she was in difficulty, went back to needing a drink.

Similarly to filling up the dinosaurs' mouths, filling up Jenny's mouth with a bottle and her stomach with water could protect against the fear of destroying or of having destroyed the mother. Repetition compulsion would again arise, as is its nature, as an attempt to master trauma and at the same time to render it visible.

When in the course of the meeting I asked something about Jenny's breastfeeding, the mother told me that it had lasted six months, and that, after a brief period of exclusively giving her the breast, this had been integrated with powdered formula. After an initial partial feeding at the breast, the little girl seemed to take the bottle well. The transition had started badly because, after five days in the hospital, the mother was discharged on a Saturday, and they had told her to give the baby a certain amount of milk with some plain cookies. The mother was very happy to have the baby home; she was overcome by the affection of relatives who, for the weekend, had not given her a "famous food supplement" (furthermore, she didn't even know what that was). At a check-up visit after the weekend, a doctor asked her almost reproachfully, "But you don't want to feed your daughter?"

This remark would continue to torment the mother for years. In any event, even though in the background she had the feeling of not being a mother up to the level of others, things had quickly gotten better. The mother liked breastfeeding her daughter, feeling that she was attached to her breast and that she sought her out, while she perceived as quite arduous the need to stick to the fixed schedule that the doctors recommended due to Jenny's poor growth rate in the early months. She did not like not being able to feed the baby on demand, as her sister-in-law had done in breastfeeding her children. She felt torn between following the paediatrician's instruction to feed her at fixed times and a rhythm that she would have felt was better. From the age of two to three months, the little girl had spontaneously skipped the night-time feeding, but the mother, in order to stick to the paediatrician's instructions, instead of adapting herself to her daughter's rhythms, had awakened her; otherwise neither of them would have awakened. Only when the baby was about three months of age did she stop doing this; the baby skipped the midnight feeding, kept the one at 3:00 a.m., and the mother awakened her at 6:00 a.m. because she had the feeling that Jenny needed more milk than what she herself felt capable of giving her. This went on until the point when, toward four months of age, they both managed to rest together for the entire night. Then, coincident with an extremely hot summer, while on vacation, the child continued to sleep calmly in her bed, and the mother, in order to protect herself from death anxiety tied to a fear of dehydration, awakened her to give her something to drink. After the summer, these maternal preoccupations about drinking ceased until the child's hospitalization at 18 months.

About eight months after the beginning of treatment, Jenny arrived at a session with her parents, punctually as usual, and once they were inside the room, she showed herself to be rather timid. According to the parents, this was in marked contrast to her strong desire to come to the appointment. As usual, the child took out some dolls and gave one to each parent, while she took care of her own doll, almost as though she wanted to reaffirm that this was a place where one looked after children's needs. The father pointed out that Jenny showed the same care and devotion that she demonstrated in her play at home, drawing on ever more symbolic attributes in playing with her dolls, imagining herself as the mom who was caring for them, going to do the shopping, etc. Then they told me that during this period, Jenny had been gladly going to day care, whereas earlier she had been bored by it. I thought that she must be one of the older children in her section, in which she would remain for some months and that she perhaps had different interests than those of her little companions. The mother agreed and explained that, even though it had been suggested to her to put Jenny in preschool, the mother didn't want to do so because it would have resulted in her going to elementary school at five-and-a-half years of age. The mother remembered the great difficulty that she herself had experienced in going to school before her sixth birthday, and – identifying with her daughter who had a medical history completely different from her own – she did not want her to suffer what she herself had suffered.

I then said that perhaps Jenny had her own ideas and needs that might not coincide with the mother's and that maybe a child who was so alert and had such pronounced skills would not have a bad experience in finding an outlet for more of her interests in a situation with children of her own age or a little older. Jenny listened to what we were saying, continuing to play. The parents continued their account of how things were going better at night, and the mother added with a mixture of satisfaction and sadness that Jenny had wanted to go to sleep at her maternal grandmother's house; she had done well there all night, without waking up. While the father emphasized that, from his point of view, these evenings should happen more often, Jenny took back her dolls, giving each person instead a little animal to play with. She found a masculine figure and gave it to her dad. Then she moved on to changing the dolls' diapers, with great skill – and imagined lovingly bathing a child who was dirty with excrement – who had asked his mom to clean up her doll as well. Then Jenny took out the big dinosaur that she usually kept a little apart, and this time, without the slightest fear, she entrusted it to the father, saying that it was "a gigantic dragon." When her father put his big masculine figurine onto the dinosaur's back, she played at "running away," saying that her doll was afraid and subsequently directing the dinosaur toward her mother, who was speaking with me, and in this way Jenny dealt with her rage toward a mother who was talking with a doctor. The session was ending, and before she left, Jenny drank some water that she had asked her father to give her. She asked her mother, "Mama, why do you drink all the time?" The question was posed in a seemingly joking way, but it provided a glimpse of the child's awareness of the mother's needs expressed through her.

A subsequent meeting with the mother and father confirmed that things were going well; the awakenings were less frequent, and the quality of Jenny's relationship with her mother was more consistent. The intensity of the mother's identification with her daughter, this time with positive aspects, could be clearly grasped when the mother said that on the weekend, they would go with the grandfather to a house in the country where she had gone for long periods as a child, and that she hadn't visited for some time.

> "I get goosebumps thinking about it!" the mother said. "I asked my father to take out all my childhood games from the cellar so that I can show them to Jenny."

All this was evidence that an identification of a healthy part of her with the child was now possible, as when she asked to "call back into service" her transitional object – imagining that, just as the little bear had helped her (at least partially) to grow up in a potential space between feeling alone, lost in unlimited loneliness, and being physically with the mother, it might be of help to her daughter as well. The reduction of split and projected persecutory fantasies in the child seemed to have made it increasingly possible to "play." This carried through in our last meeting before summer vacation, almost a year after our first contact; it was the last day of Jenny's attendance in day care, since next year she would go to preschool. While Jenny seemed not to give much weight to this, for the mother, it was a very critical moment: "Yesterday I ran out of the last meeting at day care because I was starting to cry," she said, "and Jenny noticed."

I then turned to Jenny, saying to both of them,

> You heard your mother, Jenny, when she said that yesterday she was very moved and also a little sad, thinking that you have finished in day care. It seems that she didn't want such a nice and intense period of life to end, and she cannot imagine that at preschool, too, you'll be able to do just as well.

Jenny sketched, continuing to play while the mother told me how Jenny asked for less to drink and slept all night without awakening, though the mother's death anxieties seemed to be only partially calmed; when she had woken up that morning and Jenny was still sleeping, she told her husband to "go see if she is alive." While the mother continued to talk about her progress, Jenny joined the discussion, saying that once she had dreamed about a bear: "He was very big and real, very real, and then another mother appeared in the shadows, one whom I didn't know; she was sort of normal." The dream having been related, Jenny took the big dinosaur that she had avoided at the beginning and that she now often used to express aggression, and she gave it to me to keep on the little table I was leaning on, almost to guarantee that I could keep it.

For her part, the mother at that moment seemed not to be able to accept the presence in the child's mind of an aggressive mama-bear, charged with anxiety, who little by little had caused "a sort of normal" mother to come out of the shadows, one whom the child didn't know. Showing that she had not grasped the importance of what the little girl was saying, the mother interjected that the child had begun to stutter.

I tried to follow the child's discourse and asked her what I should do with the dinosaur, who scared me a little. Then she told me that we could put it a little farther away, near the dolls' house. I said, "I wonder how afraid the dolls are when they see it, a little like what happened to you when you saw the bear." While Jenny agreed, the mother reconnected with the emotional elements of the session and said that now, when Jenny needed to, she would get out of her bed and go to her parents' bed, something that she didn't used to do because she was afraid. And Jenny remembered to specify that: "There were shadows that seemed to be a bear; there was a bear with a little flower." I remembered the fear of ghosts that she imagined were the garments on the clothes stand, and the mother remarked, surprised, that she had taken away the clothes from the stand, and now there was only a little flower on it, which had come from a wedding favour, and given that it made her afraid, she should take that away, too.

Then Jenny provided proof of her growing cognitive skills, asking me if I knew what a "black-out" was. She told me she had learned in a children's cartoon that "it is a man who takes the light for himself when there isn't any." Then she asked me if I knew what a museum was, and again in the same vein, she told me she had learned that it is a place where there are "dinosaurs and clothes belonging to princesses." In effect she was trying to show how difficult it was to rest and to move about in a place populated by voracious dinosaurs, carriers of their own aggression and of the mother's, where clothes belonging to princesses – the ghosts of the mother's past – contributed to making the place dangerous and inhospitable. Luckily, she could then dream about a bear who was not too dangerous and about a different mother whom she was learning to know.

We were at the beginning of summer vacation and exactly a year had passed since the child's hospitalization and nine months since the beginning of the sixteen meetings that had made up our work together.

The mother asked about continuing meetings with me, even though now things were going better: "We are a different couple, my husband and I, since we started coming here. We've reached many goals; even though things have a seesawing way of proceeding, thanks to coming here, I've gotten used to this seesaw."

She talked with her husband and they agreed that, given his difficulty with work – and at any rate, he had always had fewer problems with their daughter – the meetings would continue with Jenny and her mother, one for both alternating with one for the mother only. After this additional sequence of meetings, given that the little girl's improvements had been solid and the mother was much more aware of how much her problems played a role in shaping her daughter's conditions, we decided to proceed with meetings with the mother alone. In the first of these sessions, while crying softly, the mother told me about a deep conviction that she said she had never communicated to anyone: that because of her succession of physical problems, her parents' separation, and the various other misadventures that had happened to her, she felt an inadmissible feeling of inadequacy – almost a certainty that it would never be granted to her to have a healthy child. As a child, the mother had been ill, and her illness had contributed to her parents' separation, while her father left and she stayed close to her depressed mother; once she was grown up, she had dared to give birth to a little girl who, connected to a fantasy of oedipal guilt, could not be anything but ill as she herself had been.

In our second individual meeting, the mother asked if she could talk to me about something that pertained to her and did not relate to Jenny, thus allowing me to understand to what degree she was taking back the emotional overload that had previously taken shape in Jenny.

Some Theoretical Hypotheses

Not many cases are described in the paediatric literature if you exclude those written about by Kreisler (1981) and by Lebovici et al. (1985), who connect poto-mania to primitive anxieties that the child tries to calm by compulsively filling the stomach.

In the course of treating Elton, Jenny, and their parents, I often found myself thinking about the possible impact on the children of sensorial experiences that could not be transformed into psychic experiences but that had remained connected to the somatic dimension. There may have been a lack of symbolization (Roussillon 1999) in which sensorial experiences could not be translated into mental representations and subsequently into words. In this way, traces of traumatic, split occurrences from the parents' history have travelled through the generations – occurrences that have stayed connected in inaccessible areas of the psyche or the body, also because they are too intense or they happened at an age in which the psychic apparatus was still being formed or was particularly vulnerable, such as those experienced by Jenny's mother when she was very little.

The fact that in the cases described, the gastroesophageal tract was involved could lead us to imagine that early relational difficulties influenced by pre-carious medical conditions had to have been deposited into the unconscious psychic lives of both the mother and the child – traces of a basic, problematic exchange in the course of breastfeeding when the mother's pleasure is necessary because the baby gives herself up to the experience of pleasure. According to Gaddini, a fundamental moment at which the basis is formed is the first experience of the relationship with the other that is deposited in the "bodily fantasies," when the self-protective drive of children meets up with mothers' adult sexuality. This is a pleasure that seeks a reflection of one's own pleasure in the other, and the flow of milk in the child's body permits the feeling of pleasure within the self. When these experiences do not take place or take place in an altered way, with the aim of safeguarding the self's sense of cohesion, there is a shift from the relationship to the feeling, in the fantasy of being able to manage the other in an autocratic way. The importance of feelings connected to the gastroesophageal tract as the place around which early feelings are organized was also emphasized by Florence Guignard (1999). She hypothesizes that the role of contact between internal and external, habitually carried out by the skin, is in some way displaced to the digestive tract – as though, in place of instinctual sensations of hunger and satisfaction, the oesophagus has become a sensitive zone around which an early, rudimentary differentiation between "inside" and "outside" is organized.

> Inextricably tied to the subject's physical survival is the function of the digestive apparatus, which will serve as a model of the survival of the psychic apparatus.
>
> [Guignard 1999, p. 133, translation by G. Atkinson]

The experience of difficulty in the distance from the mother seems to be further darkened by a possible failure of the transitional function that leads to the emergence of the "thing-ness" of the object, to the detriment of its function, making it become a fetish, an "object regarded with awe as being the embodiment or habitation of a potent spirit or as having magical potency" (www.dictionary.com/browse/fetish). When the experience of the transitional object – the *first not-me possession* (Winnicott 1953) comes to be crystallized in a fetish and therefore compromised, it makes recourse to the bottle, to water, the equivalent of "possessing the mother."

I found myself thinking of Eugenio Gaddini's (1981) *psychophysical syndromes*. With this term, he describes a *pathology of the mind relative to detachment and separation* – in this case, a defensive syndrome that utilizes the incorporation of liquids, the oesophageal passage ("it is good," Jenny emphasizes, caressing her trachea after having drunk), utilizing a mechanism of *primitive imitation*. Primitive imitation, according to Gaddini, allows the child to restore the bodily experience with the other that is interrupted and that preserves a memory, becoming the other and reactivating that memory not only on the mental level but also in a bodily way, to re-create the experience of nourishment on a concrete level, almost as though to protect the self from intolerable detachment.

Gaddini hypothesizes that fantasies about the body may pre-date visual fantasies, and their expression in somatic terms tends to reinstate those feelings that the mind has experienced – of which it carries a memory, but these memories are maintained in the mind in an unintegrated state.

Jenny's clinical story and the changes that were evident can be read in the light of Gaddini's (1981) words:

> One can see that a psychophysical syndrome, arising in early childhood and lasting all one's life, can at times disappear during analysis, due not so much to pertinent interpretations that we provide as to the fact that the analytic process has been capable of reconstructing a mother-child situation in which certain natural processes and certain experiences, over time blocked by circumstances, have been set in motion and were allowed to happen for the first time. The impression one has is that the psychophysical syndrome disappears simply because it is no longer necessary. Its disappearance is not accompanied by anxiety about loss of the self, but one could say that it is a product of the reduction of that anxiety.
>
> [p. 513]

References

Faimberg, H. (2006). *The Telescoping of Generations. Listening to the Narcissistic Links Between Generations*. London: The New Library of Psychoanalysis.

Fraiberg, S., Adelson, E. & Shapiro V. (1975). Ghosts in the nursery: A psychoanalytic approach to the problems of impaired infant-mother relationships. *J. Am. Acad. Child. Psychiatry*, 14(3):387–421.

Gaddini, E. (1981). Early defensive fantasies and the psychoanalytical process. In *A Psychoanalytic Theory of Infantile Experience: Conceptual and Clinical Reflections*, ed. A. Limentani. London: Institute of Psychoanalysis, 1992.

Guignard, F. (1999). *Au vif de l'infantile*. Lausanne: Delachaux et Niestlé.

Kreisler, L. (1981). *L'enfant du dèsordre psychosomatique*. Paris: Privat.

Lebovici, S., Diatkine, R. & Soulé, M. (1985). *Traité de psychiatrie de l'enfant et de l'adolescent*. Paris: Presses Universitaires de France.

Roussillon, R. (1999). *Agonie, clivage et symbolisation*, Paris: Presses Universitaires de France.

Winnicott, D. W. (1953). Transitional objects and transitional phenomena – a study of the first not-me possession. *Int. J. Psychoanal.*, 34:89–97.

Chapter 9

Early Adolescence and Somatic Functional Disturbances[1]

Somatic functional disturbances – or somatoform disturbances – consist of a heterogeneous group of somatic conditions that are inexplicable from a medical point of view and that present with a certain frequency to primary care doctors or hospital wards (Luyten et al. 2012).

In the field of paediatrics, these disturbances are expressed in serious forms of bodily weakness that interfere with children's control of their legs and that cause a fear of pronounced forms of neurodegenerative pathologies, with recurrent abdominal pains, respiratory disturbances, or episodes of paroxysmal and persistent cough that by day have disabling effects and by night mysteriously disappear (Schulte and Peterman 2011; Campo and Fritz 2001). Over time, our paediatric colleagues have developed and refined a special sensitivity that leads them to raise questions about possible causes or pre-existing emotional causes in these symptomatic pictures, thereby avoiding getting to the bottom of the medicalization that often leads to a worsening of the situation.

In the face of these clinical pictures that at first glance would seem to play out exclusively on the somatic level, nowadays we try not to underestimate the symptomatic variety with which preadolescents and adolescents use the body to express "their own discomforts and their own inner conflicts when the psychic apparatus cannot successfully cope with increased drive pressure" (Blos 1962; translation by G. Atkinson).

Patients with these conditions are often referred to paediatric inpatient settings where, through joint work carried out by paediatricians and psychologists over time, one learns to take into account the complex somatic-psychological vicissitudes at an age in which an imbalance between the quality and the intensity of new impulses – and the capacities to keep them integrated into a consistent system of mental functioning – may be expressed via physical symptoms (Gutton 1991; Birraux 1993; Cahn 1998).

Valeria

A 12-year-old girl with an athletic physique, pretty and slender, has been hospitalized for a week. Tests did not reveal any organic pathology. Two weeks before

DOI: 10.4324/9781003252238-10

hospitalization, she had begun to feel tired and to have the feeling that her legs were no longer supporting her.

Early meetings with Valeria find her seated in a wheelchair while she continues to talk about extreme weakness, due to which she fears falling from one moment to the next. It's a feeling that contrasts with her athletic appearance and the way that she defines herself:

> I am very lively; I want to do lots of things. I'm nice, I have many friends, I eat a lot, and I'm very attached to my things. I'm the fastest in my class, I even beat boys in races, and I am the best in gymnastics; I'm very athletic.

Here Valeria seems to demonstrate that at this age, the development of the ego, superego, and ego ideal and psychosexual development are proceeding at different rates and rhythms. Laufer and Laufer (1984) remind us of the complexity in adolescence of integrating one's own sexed body into the self-representation.

The legs that don't support her can represent a compromise symptom with respect to conflicts between various psychic demands and fantasies connected to nascent sexuality and the oedipal dimension. With the push of pubertal development, the dismantling of the system of mental representations that was constructed in childhood seems to force the adolescent's ego into an enormous effort to withdraw from the conflict between the desire to be free of oedipal objects, on one hand and the still-present fascination with the primary love object, on the other (Ruggiero 2011, 2016).

In talking about her family life, Valeria mentions a maternal aunt who died when she was seven or eight; she remembers that her aunt had played with her, and that her mother had felt very down about missing her. She says that her parents argue frequently and that she feels closer to her father because her mother is often in a sad mood.

The fact was that the increasingly elaborate testing Valeria had undergone had not revealed clinically meaningful factors. When her discharge was outlined, her father had begun to ask insistently what was wrong with his daughter, and he had been referred to a meeting with me. His initial tone, demanding and irritated about Valeria's long hospitalization that had not led to concrete results, quickly changed to a more collaborative attitude when I told him that the exams didn't indicate any organic cause, and that – as often happens at Valeria's age – there could be emotional issues related to growing up that were being expressed via the body.

The request for an exact answer directed to a hospital delegate has quickly been transformed into a shared problem that we can confront only in collaboration. This change of observational perspective that aims at highlighting and assigning value to parental skills has suddenly and unexpectedly shifted the conversation from the limited area of somatic symptoms to spaces that are open to underlying family and intergenerational dynamics.

The adolescent development of sons and daughters constitutes a growth experience for parents, who witness their personal equilibrium put to the test – especially if the son's or daughter's encounter with adolescence reactivates unresolved emotional conflicts in the parent's own personal history and in the mixture of experiences that, starting from early infancy and on through the various developmental stages, leads the individual to become, in turn, a parent.

Valeria's mother had a sister who, at the same age that Valeria is now, became gravely ill, and after eight long years, she passed away. Valeria's mother was well aware that her sister wouldn't make it, but her relatives, in order to protect her from pain that they believed would be too great, denied the enormity of the problem. At a distance of many years, the mother carried inside the feeling that her premonitions had not been taken seriously, and now she feared reactivating the same experience with her own daughter. This time, however, she didn't want to relive the feeling of impotence that she had suffered when her fears about her sister's health had been negated and her pain had not been recognized. Now, through a repetition of the traumatic experience, which – like all repetition compulsions – brings an attenuated repetition of the experience of trauma and an implicit hope of a different result, the aim is to protect against the pain and grief of losing the sister, whose place the daughter seems to have taken. If she had taken care of her daughter, Valeria would not have encountered the same unlucky fate that struck down her sister.

This is one of the reasons behind Valeria's mother's psychic difficulty in containing her daughter's adolescent tensions, and this has probably complicated their relationship since Valeria's early childhood. At the beginning of the adolescent journey, with the unfolding of pubertal sexuality, the precariousness of the narcissistic organization that until then had supported her seemed to reveal a fragile point in the girl's psychic development. This fault line in her early development again came to light, while simultaneously offering a new chance to master it.

Identifying the daughter with the gravely ill sister seemed to express Valeria's mother's "encrypted" grief, maintained in a secret part of internal space in order to hide the pain of a loss that she could not recognize or work through (Abraham and Torok 1978). From her point of view, Valeria, through her symptomatology, found herself having to defend a narcissistic balance that was being put to the test by drive development and her new opportunities for object investment.

In fact, it is necessary to recall that the counterbalance between narcissistic investments and object investments (Jeammet 1992) – a crucial nodal point of adolescence – can in itself lead some preadolescents to register drive investment as a risk to the fragility of the narcissistic base and consequently to the processes of subjectivization (Cahn 1998).

Antonia, a preadolescent girl, effectively expressed this problem through a drawing in which she depicted herself balancing on a rope that ended in empty space, suspended over the fire of a blazing instinctuality and swaying under the pressure of the windy gusts of puberty's drives and the criticisms of a judgmental, superego-ish snake partly covered with scales, which threatened her, hissing that she "should have gotten a bad grade."

Some Theoretical Hypotheses

The definition of somatic functional disturbances includes clinical configurations based on different theoretical constructions. Bucci's (1997) multiple code theory (see also Moccia and Solano 2009), for example, represents an original contribution involving identification of symbolic and subsymbolic codes linked by referential connections at different levels of integration. According to Bucci, somatizations could be due to somatic representations that were subsymbolically dissociated or never connected to symbolic representations.

Fonagy et al. (2010) placed emphasis on the reflective function and the capacity to recognize one's own emotional life and that of others (mentalization), which derive from parental capacities to be attuned to their children's emotional states, promoting affect regulation and the ability to recognize one's own emotional states and others'.

Luyten et al. (2012, 2013) hypothesize that functional somatic disorders may be rooted in the theory of attachment or of mentalization, in close relationship with the systems that regulate stress, the immune system, and pain.

These hypotheses, together with contributions from the neurosciences, illuminate the *mysterious leap from the mind to the body* (Deutsch 1959), but in order to orient ourselves in this delicate area, it is still useful to refer to Freud's original hypotheses. Reflections on actual neuroses and psychoneuroses (Freud 1894) are still an excellent departure point for these situations that, starting from a transitory tendency toward adolescent hysteria, move on to become symptomatologies that are more directly neurotic, eventually arriving at the most complex psychosomatic symptomatology.

According to the Freudian model of après-coup, the development of sexuality during puberty can imbue the earlier blossoming of child sexuality with new meaning, and adolescence can bring with it a disposition toward hysteria:

> Although it does not usually happen in psychical life that a memory arouses an affect which it did not give rise to as an experience, this is nevertheless something quite usual in the case of a sexual idea, precisely because the retardation of puberty is a general characteristic of the organization. Every adolescent individual has memory-traces which can only be understood with the emergence of sexual feelings of his own; and accordingly every adolescent must carry the germ of hysteria within him.
>
> [Freud 1895b, p. 356]

Situations like Valeria's are placed between the "actual" and the "neurotic," in a common condition having little mental elaboration (de Ajuriaguerra 1974; Cramer 1977; Kreisler 1981; Lebovici et al. 1985). There are various opinions about the opportunity to use the terms *neurosis* and *hysteria* in the developmental phase. Campanile (2000) speaks of *hysteria of transition*, identifying as its principal characteristic a *representative deficit*, seen when the preadolescent seems not to have the representational skills that this period of his life would require. Particularly in a phase such as early adolescence, the drive's push represents an excessive quantity for the ego, which causes these drive exigencies to assume characteristics that approach the experience of trauma (Donabédian 2012).

It is very difficult to distinguish with clarity in what way somatization is differentiated from conversion. Taylor (2003) tried to confront this issue by asking whether these are effectively two distinct diagnostic entities or are in fact different terms with which to define the same psychogenetic process. He tried to individuate – as a distinctive trait between the two forms – a possible skill of the patient in expressing his story through conversion symptoms, while somatization is seen as the result of an emotional dysregulation in early childhood that approaches psychosomatic disturbances (Marty et al. 1963).

If conditions like Valeria's are understood in Freudian terms of the first topographical theory, in which the push of the adolescent drive constitutes an "excess" of excitation with traumatic characteristics, situations that are framed more directly in psychosomatic terms – such as in the case I will describe next – require an integration with the later elaborations of the second topographical theory, in which the role of the object becomes increasingly primary.

We owe much to the researchers at the Institut Psychosomatique de Paris, if the metapsychological discussion can be extended to psychosomatic symptoms as well. Since the time of the early pioneering works by Pierre Marty, Michel Fain, Michel de M'Uzan, Leon Kreisler, and their successors, Claude Smadja and Gèrard Szwec, and – pertaining to adolescence – by Diran Donabèdian, much ground has been gained in throwing light on the complex situations under discussion here.

Luisa

Luisa is fifteen years old, and for two years, she has undergone testing to try to find an organic reason for the profound astenia (weakness) that hampers her in carrying out the normal activities of everyday life – such as going to school – and at times leads her to remain in bed for an entire day. Every now and then, she runs into a doctor who believes he has found a way to explain her difficulties, subjecting her to invasive exams that inevitably lead back to the starting point.

Luisa is the third born in her family, with a brother eight years older and a sister who is the eldest of the three, described by her parents as sociable and positive, and of whom Luisa seems to be the opposite. Luisa is timid, in fact – a calm girl who does well in school and is selective in her friendships. Since she was little, she has expressed a proclivity to anticipate growth stages; for example, at one year of age, she had already established complete control of her bowel movements. From her parents' stories, it seems that the first year of her life was a problematic period, however, because the child would not let herself be held. She nursed at the breast as much as was sufficient, and immediately afterward she pulled away from her mother.

These relational difficulties seemed to be attenuated after that period, but even later on, when she accepted being held in an adult's arms, it was always contact "in small doses," which foretold a certain distance from the other. Weaned at around eight months, she had been partially bottle-fed until she was one year old, when she had stopped eating baby food because she wanted to eat like her older sister did.

The fact that – according to her parents – Luisa had never felt herself to be a child indicates a condition that Fain (1971) defined as *prematurity of the ego*, in which the little one cannot undergo the experience of passivity and trust to the care of an object. In these situations, Khan (1963) speaks of a cumulative trauma that involves a lack of maternal functions in protecting the child from too much intense stimuli or is otherwise deficient and that can lead to "premature and selective ego development. Some of the emergent autonomous functions are accelerated in growth and used in defensive action to deal with the impingements that are unpleasurable" (p. 298).

I found myself hypothesizing that a crack in early maternal containment may have led to inadequate organization of the ego's primary narcissistic foundation. This may have caused an important relational closure to occur in Luisa, who after the first year of life found an emotional balance that the development of puberty shook to its foundations.

I had arrived at one of the typical clinical situations characterized not by what is but by what is missing, in which, at a countertransferential level, I had the impression of feeling emotions in my patient's place. The absence of fantasied elaborations seems to have been well described by the concept of *operative thought* (Marty et al. 1963) – a concept that has some affinity with that of alexithymia (Nemiah and Sifneos 1970). In the latter, the patient, pressed into a dimension of superficial and factual discourse with the aim of keeping a traumatic condition at bay, seems not to possess the vocabulary or grammar of emotions, with a more-or-less marked deterioration of structures of meaning.

The absence of a "positive" symptomatology seemed to emphasize the rigidity of an archaic defensive system hidden behind a subsequent developmental journey that appeared to be harmonious enough. The girl's "negative" symptomatology, as well as an early relationship with a mother who couldn't count on a solid identification with her own mother, left room to hypothesize the presence of an *essential depression* (Marty 1966), which was evident when the psychic work connected to the transformation of drive investments came into play. Essential depression – or *depression without an object* – is characterized by a *libidinal descent without any economic counterbalance* (Smadja 2001). It is rooted in a system of early relationships dominated by ruptures in connection, still in a state of nondifferentiation between the child and the object, one in which object loss is not distinguished from narcissistic loss.

The characteristics of this type of psychosomatic disturbance have their origins in an early developmental stage. Frequently, within a mother-child relationship in which the management of sensorial exchanges has been missing, auto-erotic sensations are registered as an unbearable threat to the ego. The impracticality of hallucinatory satisfaction of desire, in the face of the object's absence, forces an investment in perceived stimuli, to the detriment of fantasy activity.

In other words, the impossibility for the child to imagine or to "hallucinate" the missing object leads to overinvesting the perceived object, in order to keep at bay the feeling of anxious impotence generated by a double loss – at the same time, both object-related and narcissistic. In this way the connections with id productions are interrupted, connections that, according to Marty (1966), *receive but do not transmit* – that is, they are not capable of transforming their contents in a way that also makes them at least partially recognizable.

In these conditions, the experience of passivity, "putting oneself into the hands of the other," would seem to be precluded, taking account only of the structuring of defences centred around a primary undifferentiated sensoriality, with the aim of excluding from the psyche all that might have any reference to the drives.

In addition to a minimal fantasied elaboration of instinctual desires, another characteristic of essential depression is the low level of symptoms and the lack of anxiety or self-recriminations. Luisa, in fact, doesn't know why she is sick. She's not anxious; she says she isn't worried about her condition because she knows she can trust her caregivers and her parents, and at any rate, if there were any problems, they would think of her welfare and take her to even better specialists.

The *psychosomatic paradox* (Smadja 2001) seems to have come heavily into play here, due to which, in the presence of an organic illness, the anxious or guilt-inducing components tend to be attenuated because the doctor becomes capable of providing interest, containment, and reassurance, which the patient and her family appear to be aware of the necessity of.

It remains to be seen why in some situations these protective systems that originate in the state of sexual development that precedes narcissistic unification – that is, the auto-erotic phase – take the form of a disturbance of emotional, relational development, and in other situations, take the form of essential depression. Luisa's case seems to point out to us an early period of life in which both possibilities were open, until a change in the relationship set the course toward psychosomatic expression.

The three nosographic concepts discussed in this chapter – actual neurosis, neurotic conversion, and psychosomatic expression – seem to be located according to the degree of access to the drive dimension and to its transformation, according to the presence or lack of a task of mental representation. It is the quality of mentalization that allows us to orient ourselves in this area, thinking of conversion as a possible skill of the patient's with which to express his or her own history through symptoms. Here actual neurosis is viewed as an excessive quantitative moment, which is also connected to the subject's temporary skills and psychosomatic symptoms as the product of an emotional dysregulation in early childhood.

Some Reflections on Working in Institutions

An emotional characteristic seen in the analyst who is coping with these situations for the first time in a hospital environment is that of an experience of considerable incomprehension.

One finds oneself in a relationship with the child's parents who, in confronting their child's conditions that often appear to be serious, look at a doctor who talks with them about emotional factors or factors pertaining to growth as though he were an extraterrestrial. Often the exchange may end up as a kind of arm wrestling in which the therapist finds himself having feelings that the patient and family tend to deny; he may be exposed to intense feelings of impotence, rejection, or incapacity and at times of rage. While to an analyst, an emotional symptom appears in relation to an organic illness within an accurate perspective, for the parents, it evokes a psychic component often equivalent to feeling themselves judged as incapable. It is therefore truly difficult for them to believe that conditions having all the traits of medical urgency, with important symptoms that often bring a child to an operating room, can be determined only by emotional variables.

The psychological approach utilized in a long-term perspective must be cautious in avoiding ill-timed proposals that can deprive future interventions of their therapeutic potentialities. Over the years, I have experienced how much, with these patients, *maintaining the continuity of the relational investment must prevail over interpretive activity* (Smadja 2001) and that, many times, the first meeting is crucial in establishing (or not) the conditions for further subsequent contacts.

In some situations, the proposal of a psychological meeting is heard with availability and a willingness to collaborate, as though the request for consultation has identified a need that was already present and awaited only an invitation to be manifested. In others – unfortunately, much more frequent – the proposal of such contact sounds like an invitation expressed in an unknown language, just as the language of affects is unknown to these individuals. There is no preclusion or rejection; the family simply lacks a vocabulary and syntax that allow comprehension of emotions. The proposed language can appear foreign, unclear, and often more worrisome than a serious organic illness.

In a *clinical situation of negativity*, to perceive unconscious dynamics at the countertransferential level – or to intuit other problems underlying the child's problems – can form the basis of "wild" interventions, which do not take account of the fact that a transformative intervention is never born of intellectual communications to someone who is not yet able to understand them.

Psychological consultation can represent an attempt to construct together with the patient a different way of posing the question, thereby transforming an unexpected and incidental meeting, wedged between an elaborate physical work-up and a medical visit, into an occasion of listening in a possible register that is different from that of the physical body.

Marty (1966) questioned why these patients come to the psychoanalyst so late. At least in paediatric practice, engaging in psychotherapeutic treatment represents the beginning of a very long and torturous journey that aims, first of all, at reconstructing the possibility of contact with emotions.

Groups

A solution I have experienced and that seems particularly versatile in the hospital environment is that of groups I have conducted with children and their parents (see the chapters on groups for parents, children, and adolescents). Group treatment has proved especially productive in those situations in which there is a difficulty in giving symbolic and communicative expression to the content that inhabits the deepest levels of emotional life. Reopening an area of faith and contact with one's own mind means to open a new flow of communication that promotes more developed states of well-being and that at times renders the experience of illness no longer necessary.

The group raises the possibility of having and sharing an experience with others who become attentive interlocutors united by their shared similar conditions and who are recognized carriers of points of view born of direct experience. The group activity brings into itself the effect of a multiplying flywheel, in that it possesses the characteristic of allowing to unfold, in very brief time periods, intra- and interpsychic emotional exchanges that in various other conditions would require much longer periods of time.

In the group, Valeria gives a shape to her primitive anxieties (Levy 2010) through the story of a dream in which she is falling. She illustrates the dream with a drawing in which she colours her lips a sensual pinkish red, thereby expressing the sexual drive that exposes her to the feeling of falling forever.

A little later, Valeria will tell about another dream, one in which she is entering a church and everyone is looking at her. In the group, a boy of about her age "interprets," helping her gain a sense of the dream through his own drawing. That drawing depicts a primitive superego with oral characteristics that observes the scene of what will come to be defined as a wedding.

In the drawing, the still-archaic characteristics of what could be a representation of the superego seem to emphasize the influence of an ego ideal that represents a narcissistic demand based on the introjection of the parents' ego ideal. From the adolescent's point of view, the presence of a demanding ego ideal makes it more difficult to recognize and hear as one's own the new thoughts, changed desires, and identity and object investments. It is only when the adolescent's ego manages to liberate itself from the impositions of the ego ideal that it can become the object of one's own narcissistic and object investments.

In leading the experience, we noticed that there was a kind of psychic permeability between parents and children or adolescents. The theoretical model that inspired us was the Bionian formulation in which the capacity for reverie allowed the transformation of elements of unspeakable anxieties, which found modulation within the group, as well as the possibility of expression and recognition. Our attempt, through a formalized group, was aimed at bringing parts of those deep emotions and sensoriality to signification and language, through what Corrao described as a *gamma function:* that is, "an unknown variable that, in the structure of the group, can be defined as a symmetrical analogy to the alpha function in an individual's personal structure" (Corrao 1998, p. 39; translation by G. Atkinson).

Only at a time a couple of years after the initiation of the group did Valeria's father recognize that some time was needed to be able to think that his daughter's physical malady could stem from something else, and it was even longer before he could accept this. He said:

> To tell the truth, at the beginning I didn't think that the group could be useful, that it could help my daughter. But now, in contrast, I think that her pains have been a unique way that she found to be able to say that she wasn't well, the only way that attracted our attention, and I must say that it has been very effective.

Conclusions

If adolescence represents for children a second moment in the process of separation-individuation (Mahler et al. 1975), then for parents, too, it is often a "third time," equally important in the stages of their life cycle. A child's difficulties can in fact represent a new chance for parents to again take up the threads of their own developmental journey, not completely finished, and, once it has been fully transited, not only will obstacles to the child's development be removed, but also the parents will be able to provide the psychic containment necessary for that development.

Hospital work inevitably leads children, parents, and us as clinical caretakers to a confrontation with mourning, that process that – beginning with the capacity to recognize the inevitable losses in relationships with our internal objects or with our body – carries us, over time, to the point of detaching from lost objects in order to find a renewed capacity to love and to establish new relationships.

When the parents arrive in our clinics, they may find themselves in a state of mourning, and their narcissism may have already been put to the test by the fact that something isn't right with their child, and an intervention of a different type than that of a medical doctor can serve almost to confirm that their parental competence is being called into question.

But we, too, as professionals are called upon to work through mourning with respect to our therapeutic ambitions (Menzies Lyth 1960), which lead us to think that our patients must stick to what we propose to them, and we feel irritated or abandoned when they do not follow our instructions and do not confirm our wish to be able to cure them. Especially in this field, great tolerance for frustration is required, as well as a deep awareness of the limits of our interventions.

Facing up to these countertransferential feelings and working through them, being at the same time present and humble in supporting our own opinions, it is necessary to keep the discussion with parents open, because providing a response to this "clinic of negativity" can have an important preventive function in relation to the consolidation of more serious pathology. And in simpler situations as well – in which, as Winnicott (1971) said, "there is only one cure for immaturity and that is the passage of time and the growth into maturity that time may bring" (p. 146) – giving support to parents and children in coping more skilfully with this particularly difficult moment has proven to be of great help in the cases I have treated.

Note

1   A modified version of this chapter appeared in the *Rivista di Psicoanalisi*, 62:463–479 (2016). The author thanks the publisher for having granted the right to republish. An English-language version was published in *The Italian Psychoanalytic Annual* as "Psychoanalysis in Hospital: Early Adolescence and Somatic Functional Disturbances" (2017).

References

Abraham, N. & Torok, M. (1978). *The Shell and the Kernel*, ed. & trans. N. T. Rand. Chicago, IL/London: University of Chicago Press, 1994.

Birraux, A. (1993). *L'adolescente e il suo corpo*. Roma: Borla.

Blos, P. (1962). *On Adolescence: A Psychoanalytic Interpretation*. New York: Free Press of Glencoe.

Bucci, W. (1997). *Psychoanalysis and Cognitive Sciences: A Multiple Code Theory*. New York: Guilford.

Cahn, R. (1998). *L'Adolescente nella psicoanalisi [The Adolescent in Psychoanalysis]*. Roma: Borla, 2000.

Campanile, P. (2000). Hystérie de transition. *Le fait de l'analyse*, 8.

Campo, J. V. & Fritz, G. (2001). A management model for pediatric somatization. *Psychosom.*, 42:467–476.

Corrao, F. (1998). *Orme. Contributi alla psicoanalisi di gruppo [Footsteps: Contributions to Group Psychoanalysis]*. Milano: Raffaello Cortina.

Cramer, B. (1977). Vicissitues de l'investissment du corps, symptômes de conversion en période pubertaire. *Psychiatrie de l'enfant*, 20:11.

de Ajuriaguerra, J. (1974). *Manuale di psichiatria del bambino [Manual of Child Psychiatry]*. Milano: Masson, 1993.

Deutsch, F. (1959). *On the Mysterious Leap from the Mind to the Body: A Workshop Study on the Theory of Conversion*. New York: International Universities Press.

Donabédian, D. (2012). *L'adolescent et son corps*. Paris: Presses Universitaires Française.

Fain, M. (1971). Prélude à la vie fantasmatique. *Revue Française de Psychanalyse*, 28:3–4.

Fonagy, P., Gergely, G., Jurist, E. & Target, M. (2010). *Affect Regulation, Mentalization, and the Development of the Self*. New York: Other Press.

Freud, S. (1894). The neuro-psychoses of defence. *S. E.*, 3.

———. (1895a). Frau Emmy von N., case histories from *Studies on Hysteria. S. E.*, 2.

———. (1895b). Project for a scientific psychology. *S. E.*, 1.

Gutton, P. (1991). *Le pubertaire*. Paris: Presses Universitaires Française.

Jeammet, P. (1992). *Psicopatologia dell'adolescenza [The Psychopathology of Adolescence]*. Roma: Borla, 2007.

Khan, M. M. R. (1963). The concept of cumulative trauma. *Psychoanal. Study Child*, 18:286–306.

Kreisler, L. (1981). *Clinica psicosomatica del bambino [Clinical Psychosomatics in the Child]*. Milano: Raffaello Cortina, 1986.

Laufer, M. & Laufer, E. (1984). *Adolescence and Developmental Breakdown: A Psychoanalytic View*. London/New York: Routledge, 2018.

Lebovici, S., Diatkine, R. & Soulé, M. (1985). *Traité de psychiatrie de l'enfant et de l'adolescent, II*. Paris: Presses Universitaires de France.

Levy, R. (2010). Adolescence: The body as scenario for non-symbolized dramas. In *Psychosomatics Today: A Psychoanalytic Perspective*, ed. M. Aisenstein, D. Rappoport & E. Aisemberg. London: Karnac.

Luyten, P. A., Van Houdenhove, B., Lemma, A., Target, M. & Fonagy, P. (2012). A mentalization approach to the understanding and treatment of functional somatic disorders. *Psychoanal. Psychother.*, 26:121–140.

———. (2013). Vulnerability for functional somatic disorders: A contemporary psychodynamic approach. *J. Psychother. Integration*, 23:250.

Mahler, M., Pine, F. & Bergman, A. (1975). *The Psychological Birth of the Human Infant: Symbiosis and Individuation*. London: Routledge.

Marty, P. (1966). La dépression essentielle. *Revue Française de Psychanalyse*, 32:3.

Marty, P., de M'Uzan, M. & David, C. (1963). *L'indagine psicosomatica [Psychosomatic Research]*. Torino: Boringhieri, 1971.

Menzies Lyth, I. (1960). A case-study in the functioning of social systems as a defence against anxiety. *Hum. Relat.*, 13(2):95–121.

Moccia, G. & Solano, L., eds. (2009). *Psicoanalisi e neuroscienze [Psychoanalysis and Neurosciences]*. Milano: Franco Angeli.

Nemiah, J. C. & Sifneos, P. E. (1970). Affect and fantasy in patients with psychosomatic disorders. *Mod. Trends Psychosom. Med.*, 2:26–34.

Ruggiero, I. (2011). Corpo strano, corpo estraneo, corpo nemico: itinerari adolescenziali tra corpo, psiche e relazione [Strange body, estranged body, enemy body: Adolescent journeys between body, psyche and relationship]. *Rivista di Psicoanalisi*, 57:823–847.

———. (2016). Il corpo ripudiato [The repudiated body]. In *La mente adolescente e il corpo ripudiato [The Adolescent Mind and the Repudiated Body]*, ed. A. M. Nicolò & I. Ruggiero. Milano: Franco Angeli.

Schulte, I. E. & Petermann, F. (2011). Somatoform disorders: Thirty years of debate about criteria! What about children and adolescents? *J. Psychosom. Res.*, 70:218–228.

Smadja, C. (2001). *La via psicosomatica e la psicoanalisi*. Milano: Franco Angeli, 2010.

Taylor, G. J. (2003). Somatization and conversion: Distinct or overlapping constructs? *J. Amer. Acad. Psychoanal. & Dynamic Psychiatry*, 31:487–508.

Winnicott, D. W. (1971). *Playing and Reality*. London: Routledge, 2005.

Chapter 10

Variations of Sexual Differentiation

Disorders of Sex Development

– "I greatly love being a woman, even against science, genetics, and destiny."[1]

During our first meeting, Renata's parents talked about their daughter's long clinical history and her problems that had led them to wander through the hospitals of central Italy. She had a masculine genetic profile, "XY," which was not congruous with her. There was a small penis, understood as a clitoris, and labio-scrotal mass with internal testes. Renata was taken for a girl at birth. No one noticed anything untoward. Even on subsequent neonatal examinations, only a general practitioner had the feeling that there was something unclear requiring further exploration.

The explorations were complex and uncertain. Between doubts, delays, uncertainties, and the fact that, as unfortunately happens in from 40 to 50% of cases, it wasn't possible to find any genetic mutation that explained the situation, some years passed.

When I first met Renata, she was almost four years old. Her parents told me that they were expecting "a miracle to happen" – that is, that the medical and psychological explorations would confirm that she was a girl, as they ardently desired, even though they couldn't hide the many sources of evidence that made her doubtful.

She was their only daughter, raised as a girl because, despite some doubts, no one until now had been able to make a diagnosis or to suggest anything different to the parents. In actuality, the initial meeting with her provoked a feeling of strangeness, given her clothes of a typically feminine type that seemed to struggle to adapt to her exuberant behaviour and her need to move about very actively.

Her parents, on the other hand, continued to see her as a little girl, even though in her play she seemed to hold herself back somewhat, and she didn't appear capable of expressing "what she really was." She preferred to be with older boys or with adults, even though when she felt secure, she played indiscriminately with boys and girls.

Sometimes she played with the dolls, but more often she behaved very actively, almost feverishly, running and jumping everywhere and making a game of every movement.

DOI: 10.4324/9781003252238-11

She had been called Renata, the name of her maternal grandmother to whom the mother had been extremely close. In the mother's view, giving her daughter the name of her own mother meant renewing the tie with her through the little girl who had been very much wished for. It seemed clear that Renata, raised as a girl, considered herself one and identified with her mother, even though the social isolation – in which the family found itself almost by choice after it was said that something wasn't right – had left them in a state of despair that could have influenced the child's development in her early years. The parents' uneasiness and desperation at the birth of a child with a possible problem in sexual differentiation were well expressed in the mother's words when she recounted having been so depressed that when she nursed the baby, she would ask herself whether she was giving her milk or poison.

Even though apparently not capable of imagining gender reassignment and all that this would mean for Renata, the parents asked themselves which would really be the better choice for their daughter. To what degree could she accept it, and how would they tell their relatives and friends about it?

A few days after our first meeting, while I spoke with the parents, a colleague began a series of observational meetings with Renata, which would be followed in subsequent years by joint meetings with the child and her parents, so that the little girl could be involved in what was being talked about.

In the sessions in which she was alone, Renata expressed difficulty in facing up to thoughts that for her were too big, unthinkable for a four-year-old. When thoughts of femininity and masculinity passed through her mind, often triggered by her play, she became rigid, gnashed her teeth, and emitted a sort of cry, hitting her head with her hands, as though she wanted to express an intolerable form of bodily sensations that couldn't be expressed in thoughts.

In the meantime, all the medical data confirmed that, setting aside the weak development of the penis and external genitals, the child's physical and biological structures were decidedly of the masculine type, and in that sense led to an inclination toward gender reassignment. The parents, following a path and a time table consonant with their needs, gradually became familiar with the idea that Renata could in effect be a little boy, and as a result they began to try to dress her as a "he," to see how they and Renata would feel about this.

It was a journey that required many months, and it reached resolution with an unexpected phone call in which the mother informed me that Renata had become Renato. The change happened suddenly, following further development of the parents' thinking; they talked to their daughter about their thoughts, and when they saw that she was calm, they felt reassured about their decision. It was not an easy decision, at any rate, because the child had a small penis, and surgery was needed to correct a urological problem.

Renato's first comment about the changed situation was simple and ingenuous in regard to the vast amount of fears and worries that required the change to be worked through. "I am a boy," he said, "and the doctors made a mistake when I was born. Now I must make myself follow along because they have to fix my willy."

One of the mother's first comments was: "All of a sudden, he's changed. He doesn't seem to be the same child any more whom I raised until yesterday – he plays soccer, he jumps, runs, and I see him liberated. We tortured him for four years."

She then added,

> The last fifteen days have been the happiest of our life. We no longer feel constrained to keep things secret, even with our dearest friends, and we have found a great deal of understanding around us. Now we feel free to have him go to the bathroom with someone else, without going along ourselves out of a fear that someone might pick up there was something strange. We didn't know how to explain it to our friends and relatives, and then we decided to speak with the parents of his school friends and subsequently with friends and relatives. We told the truth – that at birth, there was an error made in gender attribution, and now that it has been understood, he is undergoing all the exams and treatments necessary to follow up on the situation.

Renato gave the impression of feeling comfortable and at ease with his new masculine identity, and this was confirmed in all the meetings that took place over the years.

Seven years after our first session, there did not seem to be anything emerging to cast the parents' decision in doubt. The decision had been made with awareness, by weighing both positive and negative aspects of the various options in order to reach a decision about what was right for their son. This was also true because, to the degree possible, they had involved him in the decision.

Now Renato is attending the final years of elementary school, and he seems to feel himself a boy in every respect. In general, his growth and development appear to be proceeding in a positive way.

This clinical vignette helps us venture into the field of DSD – Disorders of Sex Development – as defined at the "Consensus" conference in Chicago in 2005. Experts from all medical and psychological disciplines gathered at this conference, as well as representatives of associations and support groups. A new terminology was proposed to replace more stigmatizing definitions that in the past referred to genital ambiguities, intersexuality, hermaphroditism, pseudo-hermaphroditism, etc. (Hughes et al. 2006), which will be described in detail later in this chapter.

Until we are able to make use of a new, agreed-upon definition, it will be inevitable that we refer to these conditions with the acronym DSD. Nonetheless, in trying to think of them as the expression of a variation, of a difference (D'Alberton et al. 2015), we are recognizing more and more the necessity of moving beyond terminology that refers to the concepts of disturbance and disorder to define an expression of biological, personal, social, sexual – and ultimately, human – identity. Theoreticians at the Consensus in Chicago maintained that DSD is not an entirely satisfactory term and that it is being used only until it is possible to identify a better one.

DSD has been thought of in the same way as any other medical condition – a word with which to define a pathological condition, like pneumonia. There is no problem saying that a person "has" pneumonia, but it isn't necessary to wander too far into the past to recall a time in which the pathology defined the subject, and the individual person came to be known by the name of his pathology or even by the number of his hospital bed.

Only a little more than ten years ago, the term DSD was identified by more progressive components of the scientific community, by professional associations and the medical field, as a term that respected the dignity of the people whom it came to indicate. Nevertheless, one can well imagine that this expression may have revealed its limits when those directly involved began not only to want to be listened to but also to aspire to a more active role in the management of this condition – which, after all, pertains to the definition of human subjectivity – and they began to use it as a predicate nominative (in linguistic terms), that is, as a noun that, when joined with a verb, defines the subject's condition. If, from a medical standpoint, the term DSD has a meaning in describing a condition characterized as a defect – a disturbance in genetic transcription or in the codification of an enzyme – this cannot but create problems when the part becomes the whole. The term ultimately defines the condition of a person who is a carrier of that defect and who reveals his personal, sexual, and social identity within the vast range of variability that characterizes the human condition. In fact, no one can recognize himself in the sentence, "I am a disturbance/disorder of sexual differentiation." Probably for these reasons, the term *intersex*, which was abandoned by the new terminology that considered it stigmatizing, is today starting to be utilized more often, especially in English, in order to define this condition in a positive sense – even though it risks creating new complications in associating DSD tout court with the many variations of the LGBTQ world (Cools et al. 2018).

What Are the Variations in Sexual Differentiation/DSD/Intersex?

Freud (1900, 1920, 1925) postulated an original psychic bisexuality, assuming that masculine and feminine psychic elements were present in every individual, and that, in the course of psychosexual development, these elements contributed to defining psychological structure and personal identity (Perelberg 2018). In effect that happens at the biological level, where for the first four to six weeks of embryonic evolution, boys and girls develop starting from a single genital tubercle – which subsequently, according to the genetic character and the influence of hormones tied to it – orients development in a masculine or feminine sense. Beginning with the union of the parents' genetic legacies, in every moment of this development (which involves billions of subsequent cellular multiplications), a problem can be verified, and in those cases the development of primary sexual characteristics ends up distributing itself along a continuum that unfolds between masculine and feminine.

DSD subsumes a vast group of congenital conditions that separately are rare but on the whole are frequent, in which the chromosomal, gonadic, or anatomical sex is atypical (Balsamo et al. 2016). Current classification is based on the genotype (46, XY DSD, 46, XX DSD, variations of the caryotype DSD), with further distinctions in terms of development of the gonads or of synthesis, action, or an excess of androgyny.

The principal forms of 46, XY DSD are gonadic dysgenesis, androgen insensitivity syndrome, and the deficit of 5 alpha-reductase. In these situations, individuals with a masculine caryotype XY develop genital equipment during embryonic evolution that is feminized, to a greater or lesser degree.

In the gonadic dysgenesis, the absence or nonfunctionality of the gonads means that the factors inhibiting feminine structures are not produced, and the process of virilization of the genital apparatus is not activated, with the consequent presence of external feminine genital attributes or of an ambiguous set-up with internal masculine organs or ones that are partially feminine.

In androgen insensitivity syndrome (AIS), the gonads are functioning, but the process of virilization cannot be set in motion or completed because the peripheral receptors cannot register the presence of masculine hormones. With a lack of 5 alpha-reductase, the enzyme that transforms testosterone is missing; testosterone contributes to the development of the testicles, the deferent vessels, and the seminal vesicles in *dihydrotestosterone*, a hormone that determines the development of the external genitals and prostate. Therefore, this lack means that individuals genetically and physiologically male are born with external feminine or ambiguous genital equipment, and they tend toward virilization in a very definitive way, given the influx of pubertal hormones.

In another category, 46, XY DSD includes as its primary condition congenital suprarenal hyperplasia, in which a genetic deficit impedes production of some hormones by the adrenal gland, and the absence of these for feedback causes, in some forms, a hyperproduction of testosterone, thereby triggering in girls the virilization of external genitals, while the internal apparatus remains feminine.

In recent years, with molecular biology, we have been able to recognize genetic factors underlying more than 50% of these conditions, while for the remainder, as in the case of Renato, that is not yet possible.

As we will see, the traditional medical approach to these topics was based on a strictly binary conception of sexuality stemming from a masculine/feminine antinomy.

Encountering DSD

My contact with these conditions occurred almost casually when I was asked to look into this situation in the context of the ward where I worked, which had a strong working tradition. Although this initial encounter occurred by chance, subsequent efforts and information reached fertile ground, given my earlier interests and experience as a child and adolescent psychoanalyst.

I had been accustomed to thinking that acquiring a gender identity is the result of a complex developmental journey that unfolds over years, one whose roots are interwoven with the parents' fantasies regarding the product of conception and pregnancy. I believed that subsequently, even with the influence of biological, psychological, and social factors, gender identity takes shape through the various phases of psychosexual growth and reaches its conclusion with the close of the adolescent period.

One of the developmental tasks to be grappled with is the formation of a personal synthesis with regard to the bisexuality of all human beings, which Freud placed at the root of his theory – a constitutional bisexuality and subsequent psychosexual development that influences object choice and object relationships and that comes into play in the process of the resolution of the oedipal complex.

With reference to sexual object choice, Freud wrote that:

> It is not for psycho-analysis to solve the problem of homosexuality. It must rest content with disclosing the psychical mechanisms that resulted in determination of the object-choice, and with tracing the paths leading from them to the instinctive basis of the disposition. There its work ends, and it leaves the rest to biological investigation.
>
> [1920, p. 148]

In "Analysis Terminable and Interminable," referring to the "great enigma of sex," he wrote that:

> We have penetrated through all the psychological strata and have reached bedrock. . . . This is probably true, since, for the psychical field, the biological field does in fact play the part of the underlying bedrock.
>
> [1937, p. 252]

Today we know more about the multifaceted bedrock. For example, we're more aware of the influence of hormones on the development of behaviours that are typically considered masculine or feminine (Friedman and Downey 2008, 2014), even though the biological determination of sexual constitution is still very much unknown (Birksted-Breen 1993).

In fact, gender identity does not appear as a monolithic construction. McDougall (1993), for example, maintains that among every individual's developmental tasks is that of accepting one's own monosexual destiny – working through our grief in regard to the wish to be able to encompass both genders, to be able to participate in the nature and physical characteristics of both father and mother, to be both masculine and feminine. McDougall tried to

> trace . . . the early elements that contribute to the origins of one's sense of sexual identity and the factors that may hinder the psychic process essential

to the establishment of a secure sense of core gender and sexual role. These include identifications to both parents and therefore require the capacity to resolve the universal bisexual and incestuous wishes of childhood as well as institute the mourning processes needed to assume one's monosexuality without neurotic, characterological or sexual distortions.

[199W3, p. 258]

First Impressions

With these theoretical tenets and with an inclination toward real listening in clinical psychoanalysis, I entered into an area of work that I wasn't familiar with. In the early 2000s, the deepening of the argument from a scientific point of view proceeded alongside meetings with the first persons who spoke to me about their conditions.

These two authoritative sources immediately engaged in conflict. While the scientific literature made reference to theories that dominated that sector at the time, namely, the work of John Money and the group at Johns Hopkins University in Baltimore (Money 1965; Money and Ehrhardt 1972; Money et al. 1955a, 1955b), the personal accounts that I listened to reflected great suffering wrapped in a sense of secretiveness. These accounts resonated with what emerged from patients' early associative voices, which at the end of the 1990s began to break through the curtain of silence.

To give an example of the atmosphere in those years, I will quote from a description of some episodes during that period.

> A colleague asks me, in the hallway outside the ward, what might be the best age to do a vaginal reconstruction for a 13-year-old girl with complete androgen insensitivity syndrome. He had to give a quick response to the girl's mother and help her locate a surgeon outside the area because, for reasons of confidentiality, the mother didn't want to contact hospitals in her own city.
>
> When I asked what the girl's needs were – what was known of her condition, what did the parents think about the issue, whether urgent surgical indications were present – the colleague couldn't tell me much, and what he did say had to do with maternal concerns around the possibility of the daughter having full sexual relationships once she became engaged.
>
> [D'Alberton 2004]

This case had some similarities to that of Karen, a girl with a form of 5-alpha reductase whose gonads had been removed at a young age. She had then immediately undergone numerous vaginoplastic interventions and had developed an attitude toward her body that rendered them useless, if not damaging; she perceived her reconstructed vagina as a foreign body, something that didn't belong to her.

Karen was the first DSD patient with whom I came into contact, and that allowed me to remember my first impressions – those that later on risked being covered over by a complex psychic defensive system, one that eventually affects everyone who works for a long period of time in contact with emotionally fraught situations.

At our first meeting, I noticed a disconnect between what I felt – the sensation of having before me a boy – and what I had been told, which was that she was a girl. My adaptation to this emotional dissonance appeared to me to be the sign of a collusive game that was involving me as well.

There was an intense exchange of emotions. I was unable to be spontaneous; I had to force myself to pay attention to what I said in order not to make mistakes by using the masculine gender. At the same time, I asked myself if my feeling about a sensorial communication of that type and an explicit communication on another level might not reflect the girl's relationship with herself, along the lines of there being "something that is known but that can't be talked about."

Sutton (1998) describes a similar situation, writing about moments in which, in consultation with a girl, he perceived a visible and auditory image of a boy, and he registered this at a physical level as a blow to the head that temporarily disoriented and shocked him.

Stoller (1968) used to quickly gauge the strength of the patient's gender identity by the pronoun that he found himself automatically using: "When I cannot feel comfortable with either pronoun, then I expect to find that the patient's gender identity has strong, visible masculine and feminine components" (p. 285).

Karen was 15 years of age; she lived in another city and believed that she had been referred to the hospital because of obesity. She had already seen a psychologist in her area, to whom she had been advised to "tell everything" – even that she did not menstruate and that she could not have children. She didn't know the real problem; she had been told that it must have to do with "glands in the ovaries that don't function, and that, because of this, they were removed." At the mere mention of this psychologist, whom she no longer wished to see, Karen burst into tears.

Her vagina had been reconstructed, but the lower part of her body didn't interest her; it was no longer her own, to the point that she didn't undress completely even when she took a bath. She hadn't followed through with the vaginal expansion manoeuvres that had been prescribed for her; at the time, this procedure was part of the therapeutic program of an intervention sometimes proposed even to very young girls. Karen agreed to proceed with the surgical visits only under general anaesthesia.

Returning to my colleague's question, Karen's situation came to my mind, and I couldn't help but ask myself about the advisability of an operation to the genitals of a 13-year-old girl carried out as though it didn't pertain to her – without knowing what was behind the parents' motivations, without involving, at least in part, the girl herself, in a surgery that inevitably and irreparably violated her physical integrity (the vaginal expansion manoeuvres) and interfered with the development of her bodily and gender identity, including her body's sensations and its internal representations.

I asked myself what the girl thought of her body, what she knew, if she was aware of the limited condition of her vagina, what were the mother's fantasies and fears about her daughter's sexual ambiguity, and what did the father think.

What would prevent intervention at a later time, when the problems had been presented and had motivated the girl to undergo surgery that would permit her to have complete sexual relationships?

Changes in Medical and Psychological Practices

At about the middle of the 1990s, persons who were directly involved began to make their voices heard through associations and support groups (www.isna.org, www.cah.org.uk), and they began to bring up for discussion what Karkazis (2008) called *the traditional treatment paradigm.*

This was a mixture of almost universally accepted rules. It was affirmed that:

- Sexual gender identity is undifferentiated, plastic, and malleable during the first 18 months of life, in both boys and girls;
- The development of sexual gender identity requires unambiguous genitals, and that implies an early normalizing surgery, possibly by the end of the second year of life; and
- The parents must not show doubts in their behaviour with their child in conforming to the assigned sex that has been decided upon.

This approach implied, as a corollary, a tendency not to give out information and to leave people in the dark with respect to their conditions.

This is a very rare condition, such that, until a short time ago, an encounter with a case of DSD was an event of extraordinary interest in professional practice for a clinician who, like me, when he tried to educate himself about it, ran into those who believed themselves to have more advanced theories or who even supported the theories expressed by Money and colleagues (Money 1965; Money and Ehrhardt 1972; Money et al. 1955a, 1955b).

A case that became emblematic was that of the Reimer twins, two homozygous boys in a remote Canadian province (Colapinto 2000). One of them incurred a tragic accident when, at seven months of age, due to a routine circumcision for a phimosis, he suffered a penile burn that required removal. After a long and desperate period, the parents heard Dr Money talk about his theories on TV and thought they had found a solution; the trip from Winnipeg to Baltimore, 2,500 kilometres, was easily dealt with in order to resolve little Brian's problems. For Money, a perfect "laboratory" situation took shape with which he could prove his theories: identical twins, one a boy and the other genetically male but raised as a girl after a bilateral orchidectomy and surgical intervention to construct a vagina. The parents were following doctors' instructions and forcing themselves not to say anything about what had occurred.

In reality, things did not go at all well, but despite some criticisms (Diamond and Sigmundson 1997), this situation was presented as an example of success for some years (Money and Ehrhardt 1972). Brian became Brenda and spent a difficult childhood as a girl who played with boys and who engaged in activities that involved wrestling, movement, and competition. At puberty, she also undertook feminizing hormonal therapy, until she began to insistently ask her father the reason for all the trips and visits to hospitals. When her dad told her the truth, for the first time, she had the feeling that things inside herself – himself – had a meaning, that the sensations he felt in his body and mind corresponded with what had been said. He stopped taking oestrogen, took the name David, and faced a new life as a boy. He turned to surgical remedies to "virilize" his genitals; he began to have affective relationships with women; but in the end the emotional charge of what had taken place, the physical conditions, perhaps even the media exposure that his case was triggering, created a situation such that, in 2004, not yet 40 years old, he took his own life.

But times were changing, and more criticisms were raised in regard to traditional treatment methods. The paternalistic attitude, through which decisions devolved primarily to doctors, became a subject of discussion, including decisions about gonadectomies, feminizing genital surgeries, the creation of a vagina by utilizing a part of the intestines with the necessary expansions, reduction of the clitoris, and maintaining secrecy "in the patient's best interest."

Most especially, the advent of the Internet allowed people who were directly involved to begin to contact each other and to share experiences, often of great suffering and loneliness, and to talk about these. One of the first ones who did so was a 63-year-old woman who wrote to the editor of a medical journal, saying that for her entire life, she had felt there was a secret inside herself. The fact of not knowing exactly what the secret was had stayed with her like a shadow of fear and had severely limited her in meeting life's challenges. Being in psychiatric treatment for some time was not helpful to her because the therapist stuck to the protocol that was then in vogue, instructing her not to tell anyone anything about her physical conditions. She wrote:

> Decades later . . . having discovered an international self-help group, a world of self-acceptance opened up for me. My great regret is not having received information and help when I was a girl. I had the psychological strength to confront my sexual ambiguity, had I been given the chance. But I didn't have the chance.
>
> [Letter to the Editor, *Canadian Medical Association Journal*, 1966, 154:568–570]

Subsequently, another individual spoke up in Dublin in 1996, at the Congress of the British Society of Pediatric Endocrinology. And in a posting on one of the first websites established by an initial Androgen Insensitivity Support group, a person told of having spent two years speaking with various professionals about the disorder but only for a total of about 20 minutes, given that the caregivers talked 99% of the time, leaving the patient to merely gesture "yes" or "no." Even less than 20 minutes were devoted to trying to speak with the parents about the problem.

After having detailed his dramatic search for meaning in what he perceived to have happened in his body, finally having found basic help in one of the early support groups, the patient concluded his comments, saying that he felt the involvement of psychologists was essential in diagnosing the disorder, as were conversations with both parents and with children and adolescents for further clarification.

From then on, things continued to change significantly, but resistances were numerous and took various forms. Money's prescriptions were considered axiomatic for decades and for generations of clinicians, due to a series of factors: the prestige and academic authority of those who put them forward, the lack of knowledge about a reality that was so rare that it didn't allow alternative opinions – and finally but not least, the fact that these reduced the complexity of the problems, forcing the issue into a narrow sexual binary of male/female, outlining something apparently simple in a field full of uncertainties.

Scardovi (2012) defined a similar attitude as *cognitive compliance:*

> From a cognitive point of view, compliance appears as the unaware tendency to assign to something outside of us, which we assume to be objective, a primacy of value and meaning that exempts us from the responsibility of contact with what we are relating to, according to a deep and unknown need for delegation. This is a limitation of our responsibility toward the other, against whom we defend ourselves out of fear of excessive contact, but on an internal level, it also expresses difficulty in allowing the self to be able to think with sufficient independence and freedom. The same word, *"com-pliance,"*[2] indicates something that has to do with pleasure, but it is not a pleasure that one wants to reach in accord with a desire. Rather, it represents an intra- and interpsychic arrangement that informs the broad human attitude toward embracing an assumption in which this promises a "certainty" to those who can tolerate it, manifesting a type of attachment in which the more there is delegation, the more one feels oneself conforming, and in which one feels "right" because of being in some way "obedient."

Something very similar happened in addressing DSD, and sometimes it still happens, because none of us is immune to inheriting the past and the methods that were proposed to protect against the impact of a reality that reactivated fantasies, fears, and conflicts.

The emotional aspects tied to DSD lead us to think of the body's concrete reality: we must be helped to construct for ourselves a more symbolic way of thinking, of going beyond the binary logic of yes/no, of the presence/absence of masculine/feminine.

Currently, one of the possible motives for which the habits of the past are slow to die is this: the encounter with DSD, considered an exception at some specialized centres, is identified as an exceptional event in most health professionals' routines. Thus, the presence of DSD reactivates fantasies, fears, and conflicts and exposes us to contact with areas of anxiety and worry. The emotional equilibrium is shaken to its foundations in health care workers and in parents, who during our early childhood allowed each of us to come to terms with primary relationships, sexual and aggressive impulses, and curiosity about childhood sexuality, making it possible for us to digest these as part of our intellectual development (D'Alberton 2010).

If we do not confront the irrational emotional factors tied to DSD, even our ability to think may be blocked. Sutton (1998) recommends that in this regard, we must be able to maintain a "capacity to think in an appropriate way" (p. 200).

In order to do that, in his opinion, it is necessary that we understand that our professional skills in this sector have developed at least in part out of the sublimation of our interests and of our childhood sexual curiosity. And the more we are free to explore and remain open to the emotional complexity connected to these topics, the more we will notice emotional resonances linked to factors that are tied to the events of our personal history and our development.

> The converse is that splitting and denial occurs – these impulses are encapsulated in an area of the mind where they cannot be used because a threat is contained in them which has to be controlled, but at a cost to the overall functioning of the individual. Mental work has to be done to maintain and keep them in their place, and experiences that might somehow incite them, giving them more force, have to be avoided.
>
> [Sutton 1998, p. 245]

An example of that can be represented by the advice often given in the past when a reassignment of gender was required: that of moving from one city to another; in other words, one shifted to the external world that which was considered unacceptable by the internal world.

This was at risk to happen in the case of Renata/Renato when the parents, after having made the decision together with Renato to proceed with a masculine identity, had initially thought of going to live in a different area, as someone had advised them to do. In the end, however, in order not to lose connections with friends and relatives, they decided to cope with their problems without moving away. As they explained:

> In the first weeks after we made our decision, we almost didn't go out of the house. When we did go out, we parked in front of the door of wherever we were going and let the child go inside quickly, out of a fear that someone would say, "But how the hell have they dressed that little girl?!" Then we thought about talking to various relatives to explain things to them. Later on,

we talked about it with friends, and subsequently we decided to talk to everyone, one by one. We went to the homes of our friends whom we would see at the park for play time and explained things to them as well. We told Renata's friends, too, that when she was born, an error had been made; it was thought she was a girl, but instead she was a boy and is now called Renato. From then on, these young friends did not use the wrong name even once. The adults asked to understand more about it, and their being close by was a great help. We needed their help in order to again feel we were part of the social group, since earlier we had experienced isolation while feeling our pain. After we talked to the first few people, word got out, and we actually met with a considerable amount of understanding as well as discretion. In our town, by now everyone knows what happened but no one says anything; at most, they ask how Renato is doing.

Awareness of One's Own Condition

When I find myself reflecting on the attribution of the right that we claim to decide what a person can or cannot know about him- or herself, I think of Annamaria, a girl with Morris syndrome, identified at age 16 following primary amenorrhea. Her gynaecologist, facing an unclear clinical condition, had asked for a chromosomal map, from which an XY karyotype emerged. Annamaria was not told anything about her situation, and when, as was standard at that time, the gonads were removed in order to avoid the hypothetical risk of a tumour, she was told that her ovaries had been taken out.

At a subsequent hospital admission, Annamaria – who was 16-and-a-half, very intelligent, had many interests, and was doing extremely well in high school – related that, even though she had cooperated with all the required assessments, she was fed up with the many medical visits. When she got close to the hospital, she would experience a panic attack. She maintained that she felt herself to have been violated regarding her basic rights because a decision had been made about her – and about her body – without her having been asked anything about it. Her pain was made more acute by her conviction that at 16, she should have been allowed to actively participate in the decision regarding surgery.

Based on the accounts of many people with DSD, it seems a given that the final stage of the developmental journey consists of the complete knowledge of one's own condition – avoiding the distractions of occasional events such as a hospital stay or a test for suspected infertility and being abruptly forced to come to terms with an unknown reality or one only barely intuited.

One might doubt whether this is actually an unknown reality, as indicated in the foregoing statement. It is more probable that there is an intervention in the form of a subtle game of defensive collusions among doctors, parents, and patients – and why not, among psychologists as well – based on a system of denial through which everyone knows everything, but they behave as though no one knows anything.

If there seems to be a definite necessity that, sooner or later, a person will become conscious and will arrive at a clear internal narrative construction about his true condition; the point is how to reach this awareness without negatively interfering with individual and social developmental processes. And we have seen in the chapter about communicating diagnoses that this is very far from necessarily constituting a traumatic experience.

If one needs further confirmation, we can turn to Brian Reimer (here called "John"), whom we met earlier, who speaks to us about how he felt when, after years of suffering, he learned how real his experience actually was:

> In an episode of crying that followed a particular exhortation on John's part, the father told him the how and why of the story that had been transpiring. John remembered: "All of a sudden everything clicked. For the first time, things made sense and I understood who and what I was."
>
> [Diamond and Sigmundson 1997, p. 4]

According to this view, drawn from clinical practice, evidence emerges that emphasizes the importance of framing the truth to patients (D'Alberton 2007).

> Children do not think as adults do. They would therefore be less worried than adults are about a diagnosis with serious or ominous implications, yet they are commonly left uninformed until someone judges that they are old enough to understand. For most, this means delivery of painful information during the very vulnerable teenage years. A better approach is to unfold the truth stage by stage, matching simple statements to the child's conceptual growth until the personal implications are finally realised as part of a maturing process.
>
> [Goodall 1991, p. 34]

Not being taken seriously, even if one's need to know is still within a childhood context, is in fact one of the most painful and secret wounds that emerge in the suffering of persons who in adult life choose to undergo psychoanalytic or psychotherapeutic treatment.

As we have said, things are changing rapidly. All over the world, associations and support groups have become the most sensitive parts of professional teams who work in this area, contributing to an extensive effort to revise methods and procedures. As in many other countries (www.dsdfamilies.org, www.dsdteens. org), in Italy in 2006, the Aisia association (www.aisia.org) is active and works in dedicated and valuable ways, as do groups of activists such as Intersexioni (www.intersexioni.it). National and international study groups have begun to debate this issue with multiprofessional initiatives and with the contribution of directly involved associations, such as the Italian study group on DSD (www. gruppodistudio-it-dsd.org).

From a practical point of view, in these discussions, controversial topics in DSD management are being explored in ever-greater depth, starting from what was established at the Chicago Consensus, which approved five principles of assistance:

1. Gender assignment must be avoided before there has been an evaluation on the part of neonatal experts;
2. Long-term evaluation and management must be carried out in a centre with a team of multidisciplinary experts;
3. Every individual must be assigned a gender;
4. Open communication with patients and families is essential, and their participation in the decision-making process should be encouraged;
5. The patient's concerns and those of the family must be respected and treated with maximal confidentiality.

Some of these points are already controversial, such as the one prescribing that all individuals must be assigned a gender. Reactions range from the position that tends toward the possibility of not declaring a baby either masculine or feminine in situations in which that is not permitted by somatic conditions, to the statement of the right not to be defined in the registry or in identity documents as either masculine or feminine – as has been confirmed by recent decisions in Germany, Australia, India, Canada, Malta, and Argentina. This is something that it is possible to do without medical certification in the state of New York (www. nbcnews.com/feature/nbc-out/gender-x-new-york-city-add-third-gender-option-birth-n909021), effective January 1, 2019, previously adopted by other states in the USA (Oregon, California, Washington, and New Jersey).

On other points, the consensus is almost unanimous (Cools et al. 2018). There is substantial agreement on the need to limit surgical interventions to those that are strictly necessary, postponing those not necessary for the health of the patient until the time that it is possible for him to express his opinion, as indicated in a recent resolution at the "Consiglio d'Europa" of 2017. This is also true because excessive recourse to "normalizing" surgery can lead to an ideological refusal of those interventions that can actually improve the quality of the person's life.

By now there is also agreement on the necessity for these conditions to be followed by specialized centres that have proven experience and can make available all the professionalism utilized to compose a multiprofessional team necessary to cope with these conditions, composed of paediatric endocrinologists and/or adult endocrinologists, psychologists, neonatologists, paediatric surgeons, gynaecologists, geneticists, molecular biologists, radiologists, etc.

The importance of the work group does not reside only in the possibility of integrating approaches stemming from diverse professions but is more especially because, when things function well, a way of thinking is activated – that of the work groups themselves, a way that is infinitely richer than the sum of the contributions of the professionals of which it is composed. In the group, concerns that every individual would have trouble keeping to himself can be expressed, containing anxieties and attempts to find "loopholes" through active interventions, and thus one can overcome emotionally difficult moments and find the strength to bear uncertainty. This is necessary in order to proceed, together with patients and/ or their parents, along new pathways.

But the multidisciplinary group is not only a technical option that differentiates better or worse interventions; it is an indispensable working modality in this field in which journalistic and judicial investigations are beginning to be more and more frequent. For example, on October 12, 2017, the BBC broadcasted a report in which the Great Ormond Street Hospital, one of the most prestigious European paediatric hospitals, was accused of not respecting the standard of care for children with DSD (www.bbc.co.uk/news/uk-41593914).

The hospital records under scrutiny pertained to the fact that direct psychological support was not available for children and families who had turned to the hospital for help, despite the continuation of surgical interventions in the previous months. The BBC ascertained that dozens of families were awaiting therapy and that, for many years, not all children and their families had had access to psychological consultation before undergoing a surgical intervention. Another record pertained to the fact that not all the cases had been adequately discussed in multidisciplinary teams.

It was stated, then, that from the moment that information on this type of pathology becomes complex and the parents are not given informative material in written form to take home, adequate comprehension was not guaranteed in a way that would enable patients to knowingly give informed consent before an irreversible surgery took place. Investigations of this type are being promoted in a more significant way all over the world, spurred on by public opinion that is beginning to put forth serious doubts about the actual wishes of health professionals to truly modify the situation.

In recent years, changes in the treatment of DSD/intersex situations have taken into account the errors of the past and have seen the persons directly affected as ever more involved in health practices that pertain to them. At the root of this new way of practicing is the individual's right to complete knowledge of his own condition and to exert full and informed consent to medical treatments, whether or not they are irreversible.

This is a complex process that, going back to the time when the problem was presented for the first time, must involve a multidisciplinary team of health workers, the parents of children with DSD, and adults with DSD. In more favourable situations, referral to a support group would be among the options of which individuals can avail themselves, because reassurance from people who have directly lived this experience is something that health professionals cannot offer. The result of a process of such complexity cannot always be replicated in a uniform way; the encounter between scientific types of knowledge and emotional factors can lead us to embark on journeys that are unpredictable at the outset. But with the shared vision of a possibility of living in harmony and in an authentic way with DSD, an integration can be achieved between biological reality and psychological reality, one that opens new possibilities for all the participants in this complex process.

Attempts to erase the reality of a body that was born different, without the agreement of the person directly involved, reflects both a great necessity to control life and an excessive fear of the uncertainty that is intrinsic to life. This denial protects us and our society from uneasiness, the uneasiness that derives from what we have always known – that masculinity and femininity are never mutually exclusive. By eliminating every possibility of an encounter between these two realities, we can reduce the fear and complexity of interventions, but in doing so we also eliminate the hope of thinking in a more open way, outside preconceived patterns.

Notes

1   Here a person speaks to the androgynous members of an Aisia support group (www. aisia.org) about his/her condition of insensibility.
2   Translator's Note: In Italian, *com-piacenza*.

References

Balsamo, A., Ghirri, P., Bertelloni, S., Scaramuzzo, R. T. & D'Alberton, F., et al. (2016). Disorders of sexual development in newborns. In *Neonatology: A Practical Approach to Neonatal Diseases*. New York: Springer, pp. 1–24.

Birksted-Breen, D., ed. (1993). *The Gender Conundrum*. London: Routledge.

Canadian Medical Association Journal (1966). Letter to the Editor. 154:568–570.

Colapinto, J. (2000). *As Nature Made Him: The Boy Who Was Raised as a Girl*. New York: HarperCollins.

Cools, M., Nordenström, A., Robeva, R., Hall, J., Westerveld, P., Flück, C., Köhler, B., Berra, M., Springer, A., Schweizer, K. & Pasterski, V. (2018). Caring for individuals with a difference of sex development (DSD): A consensus statement. *Nature Review/ Endocrinology*, 14(7):415–429.

D'Alberton, F. (2004). Le ambiguità genitali, riflessioni sul trauma, sul segreto, sul dolore e sull'integrazione [Genital ambiguities, reflections on trauma, on the secret, on pain and on integration]. *Psichiatria dell'infanzia e dell'adolescenza*, 71(4).

———. (2007). Telling stories, telling lies: The importance of a progressive full disclosure of SDS. Paper presented at ISHID II World Congress on Hypospadias and Disorders of Sex Development, November 16–17, Rome. www.aissg.org/PDFs/D'Alberton-ISHID-Rome-2007.pdf.

———. (2010). Disclosing disorders of sex development and opening the doors. *Sex Dev.*, 4:304–309.

D'Alberton, F., Assante, M. T., Foresti, M., Balsamo, A., Bertelloni, S., Dati, E. & Mazzanti, L. (2015). Quality of life and psychological adjustment of women living with 46, XY differences of sex development. *J. Sexual Med.*, 12:1440–1449.

Diamond, M. & Sigmundson, H. K. (1997). Sex reassignment at birth: Long-term review and clinical implications. *Archives Pediatrics & Adolescent Med.*, 151:298–304.

Freud, S. (1900). The interpretation of dreams. *S. E.*, 4/5.

———. (1920). The psychogenesis of a case of female homosexuality. *S. E.*, 18.

————. (1925). Some psychical consequences of the anatomical distinction between the sexes. *S. E.*, 19.

————. (1937). Analysis terminable and interminable. *S. E.*, 23.

Friedman, R. C. & Downey, J. I. (2008). Sexual differentiation of behavior: The foundation of a developmental model of psychosexuality. *J. Amer. Psychoanal. Assn.*, 56:147–175.

————. (2014). Sexual differentiation of childhood play: A contemporary psychoanalytic perspective. *Archives Sexual Behavior*, 43:197–211.

Goodall, J. (1991). Helping a child to understand her own testicular feminisation. *Lancet*, 337(8732):33–35.

Hughes, I. A., Houk, C., Ahmed, S. F. & Lee, P. A. (2006). Consensus statement on management of intersex disorders. *J. Pediatric Urology*, 2:148–162.

Karkazis, K. (2008). *Fixing Sex: Intersex, Medical Authority, and Lived Experience*. Durham, NC/London: Duke University Press.

McDougall, J. (1993). The dead father: On early psychic trauma and its relation to disturbance in sexual identity and in creative activity. In *The Gender Conundrum*, ed. D. Birksted-Breen. London: Routledge.

Money, J. (1965). Psychological evaluation of the child with intersex problems. *Pediatrics*, 36:51–55.

Money, J. & Ehrhardt, A. (1972). *Man and Woman, Boy and Girl: Differentiation and Dimorphism of Gender Identity from Conception to Maturity*. Baltimore, MD: Johns Hopkins University Press.

Money, J., Hampson, J. G. & Hampson, J. L. (1955a). Hermaphroditism: Recommendations concerning assignment of sex, change of sex, and psychologic management. *Bull. Johns Hopkins Hospital*, 97:284–300.

————. (1955b). An examination of some basic sexual concepts: The evidence of human hermaphroditism. *Bull. Johns Hopkins Hospital*, 97:301–319.

Perelberg, R. J., ed. (2018). *Psychic Bisexuality: A British-French Dialogue*. London: Routledge.

Scardovi, A. (2012). Chi ha paura del piacere? Etica e sessualità nel lavoro di cura [Who is afraid of pleasure? Ethics and sexuality in the task of curing]. Paper given at Psychoanalytic Center of Bologna, April 12.

Stoller, R. J. (1968). *Sex and Gender: The Development of Femininity and Masculinity*. London: Routledge, 1994.

Sutton, A. (1998). "Lesley": The struggle of a teenager with an intersex disorder to find an identity – its impact on the "I" of the beholder. In *A Stranger in My Own Body*, ed. D. Di Ceglie & D. Freedmann. London: Karnac.

Chapter 11

Group Therapy with Parents, Children, and Adolescents

Over the years, a group of my colleagues came together, clinicians who visited the hospital for various reasons and who worked in different areas of the hospital. Sometimes they were there to complete postgraduate training or specialty programs; some had scholarships or contracts with varying schedules, and some visited for specific projects and more structured activities.

Commonalities in training and in scheduling led to a weekly meeting that gathered together on average about 15 colleagues. As these meetings proceeded, we often found ourselves reflecting on the experiences we had already set in motion with personal groups or with doctors in training, and the idea of experimenting with group activities gained more and more traction.

We saw the importance of group work early on in its effects on us. Our meetings became actual "compensation rooms" for emotions, thoughts, and curiosity, born of a variety of clinical situations, which were enriched and transformed in a frequently surprising way, thanks to our colleagues' listening to each other and their contributions.

Over the years, the "Monday meeting" became a time of theoretical focus and clinical comparisons – an incubator of projects and a builder of strong relationships. In that meeting, people took turns presenting the activities they were conducting at various levels – the conversations, testing results, psychotherapeutic sessions, and discussions of new projects.

We found ourselves talking about groups more and more often, again thanks to the skills of some of the colleagues whose experience had already matured or who had specific training in that field. The idea of therapeutic journeys conducted with groups of children, adolescents, and parents seemed ever more appropriate for providing answers to the therapeutic questions that were often directed to us and to which we couldn't always respond with the classical tools of individual interventions. Already in our early preparatory activities, we saw evidence of how the group experience allowed for emotional exchanges to unfold among the participants, which under different conditions would have required a much longer time to emerge.

Beyond sharing our experiences, we were able to enhance our knowledge of groups from a theoretical point of view. Then, with the support of an association,

DOI: 10.4324/9781003252238-12

we embarked on a monthly supervision program for some years with Anna Baruzzi, a psychoanalyst with special expertise in conducting groups. Our subsequent experiences confirmed how much the group experience carries within it the effect of a multiplying flywheel for the working through and transformation of psychic experiences.

The theoretical model that inspired us was the Bionian one, according to which the group's mental apparatus allows transformation of unthinkable anxieties, through which modulation and the possibility of expression are achieved. On the basis of experiences that took place during and immediately after the Second World War, Bion (1961) began to experiment with a personal way of working with groups, and he noticed that the group expressed its own fantasies around the stated objectives. In this way he identified a *group mentality*, which defined the group as a unified whole endowed with a *group mind*, a common reservoir into which the contributions of all the members poured in, even though they had no awareness of it; indeed, while the individual might in some way be opposed to it, at the same time he contributed to forming it.

The group mentality is distinct from the *group culture*, or rather from the structure that the group creates for itself over the course of its development, according to its objectives. In this view, the group is characterized as a separate entity, distinct from the whole of the individuals who comprise it. The group is permeated by fantasies that catalyse emotional life, fantasies that can assume psychotic characteristics and tend to be repeated with unconscious group defensive mechanisms.

Through these mechanisms, anxieties tied to group participation are expressed with a modality defined by Bion as *basic assumptions:* namely, *pairing, fight/ flight,* and *dependency.* According to Bion, the ceremonies and formalities of the aristocracy and of institutions could be an expression of the basic assumption of pairing, and in them one could see in action the basic assumption of fight/flight, while that of dependency characterized the relationship with superior entities, such as the State or the Church. Achievement of the group's rational objectives occurred because of the construction of a *working group* in which various basic assumptions were combined, overcome, and expressed in a more balanced way.

Through the experiences that unfolded within it, over time, a group could transition from a way of functioning according to basic assumptions to more of a work group functioning.

Groups with Parents

Early activities pertained to the parents of children who periodically entered the hospital for chronic conditions that had to be followed and monitored over time. The mother of one young boy asked me what would be the optimal age at which to send a child alone to a summer camp that was designed to foster autonomy and socialization for preadolescents with diabetes. We were at the fifth of a series of eight meetings arranged for young children, those under ten or eleven years of age. The meeting had yet to begin; most of the parents were already seated and were talking about things that appeared extraneous, but that we had learned to recognize as unconscious contents that would then become issues that the group would address within the "formal" frame.

When I answered the woman by saying that we could talk about this together, she replied with conviction, "Yes, all right, we'll chat about it."

The idea of referring to verbal and emotional exchanges that had happened in earlier meetings as "chats," far from devaluing what had happened, reflected the progressive lightening of emotional intensity that characterized the way in which parents addressed the topics that they decided to bring in.

That early experimental group had been launched with the parents of children with diabetes because, in periodic individual meetings that we had had with them, it seemed to us that we were encountering tremendous suffering and an unmet need to relate to others.[1] As in other situations in which routine visits didn't seem to reveal specific problems, we noticed a need to address the emotional aspects connected to chronic illness that arose suddenly during childhood or adolescence. Together with colleagues who were expert in the area of diabetes, we tried to avoid managing the illness in a way that often ended up limited to its "technical" dimension, almost out of a necessity to protect against contact with emotions.

It has been written that diabetes is an illness "difficult to live and difficult to think" (Cramer et al. 1979). In our experience with children, we have had continuing confirmation from youngsters and their parents of how difficult it is to make sense of and to explain to one's self and others, a condition like diabetes that escapes exact definition. Which zone of the body it concerns is not well understood; it originates in the pancreas but pertains to a great number of bodily organs. It is connected to medical treatment but also to nutritional habits and patterns of movement; too much sugar in the blood leads to problems, but too little blood sugar is also problematic.

The problem encountered at the onset of a chronic illness is that of finding ways for a potentially traumatic event to be integrated and mentally elaborated by the person who must live with his family members in such a way that, over time, the risk diminishes of the emergence of very intense expressions of suffering that mobilize defensive, self-protective mechanisms that do not promote integration or psychic maturation (D'Alberton et al. 2012).

The onset of diabetes interrupts the silent dialogue in the relationship between body and mind. Children and their families must find a new equilibrium that takes into consideration both practical management and the emotional aspects connected to it. A tendency to separate physical aspects from psychological ones is often seen. Sometimes doctors tend to assign relative importance to the patient's emotional life, and psychologists may neglect aspects that are closely linked to the body. In our work, we have tried to examine the dynamics tied to the onset of diabetes and to evaluate the degree to which un-worked-through emotions can influence psychic equilibrium and the patient's capacity to continue in therapy. We have therefore tried to develop some of the ideas that Fonagy and Moran (1993) expressed around "the presence of irrational anxieties rooted in the unconscious, personal meaning of some aspects of the diabetic realm" (1993, p. 65), with the hope of coming up with a more complete treatment for this chronic illness through integration of somatic aspects with psychic ones (Fonagy and Moran 1993).

Together with colleagues who are specialists in diabetes, we therefore arranged psychodynamically oriented group meetings aimed at parents, in which to compare and explore parental topics. The goal was to facilitate expression and recognition of emotions, with particular attention to those connected to or aroused by diabetic illness and insulin therapy.

Practically speaking, we hoped that the groups would promote greater familiarity with emotional elements related to the presence of diabetes in order to be able to verbalize difficult or conflictual aspects of the treatment, to give a name to feelings, to distinguish what was real from what was an expression of fantasies about what diabetes involves, differentiating the children's emotional difficulties that had to do with this illness from those that pertained to the physiological stages of their development. In addition, the groups tried to encourage sharing and expression of the real emotional burden of the experience of parenting a son or daughter with diabetes.

An aspect we were curious about was the attempt to determine up to what point there was a kind of psychic permeability between psychological work with the parents and the experiences that children and adolescents were living out in their relationship with them. At times, those relationships were transformed according to a changed perspective on some of their psychological difficulties, and we noted empirically that these changed perspectives of earlier experiences were associated with an improvement in metabolic parameters. For example, six months after the first parental group was initiated, the glycaemic haemoglobin of children whose parents participated in the group had gotten worse in two cases but improved in all the others.[2]

Of course, these were casual results that did not meet the criteria of objective validation of a medical intervention, but they inspired us to draft a project that would adhere to scientific research protocols, hypothesizing a randomization of group experiences in order to be able to examine possible correspondence between psychological variables/quality of life on the one hand and metabolic parameters on the other. Unfortunately, the precarious nature of the organizational situation of our group didn't allow us to carry the project to completion, given that it would have required a more stable temporal and managerial dimension than we could offer.

The formation of groups came about through a letter sent to the parents of children followed at our clinic. The positive responses allowed us to initiate two groups, one for parents of the youngest children and the other for parents of those who attended middle school and high school.

The groups were led by a psychologist-psychoanalyst, an expert in diabetes and an observer. The meetings did not have a specific theme or agenda but left open to the parents the opportunity to talk about whatever aspect of their experience they wished to bring to the group's attention. Each meeting lasted 1 hour and 45 minutes;

meetings were held every two weeks in repeatable cycles of 8 sessions. Both the length of each meeting and the number of sessions had been decided by taking into account factors determined by the administrative and organizational rules at the institution, in addition to our knowledge of conducting groups. For example, our consideration of the optimal sequence of sessions reflected the fact that, for administrative reasons, each medical prescription permitted a maximum of eight administrations of treatment, hence the eight-session sequences. Our efforts were successful in creating an environment that allowed parents to express themselves so that we could confirm the validity of our intuitions.

"This is the first time that I'm talking about this to anyone, and I'm doing it because I know I'm with people who know what I'm talking about" – these were the first words from a mother who, between bouts of crying, opened the first meeting. This emotion was shared and reinforced by all the other parents in an atmosphere of being very deeply moved, one in which the levels of pain reached the limits of what could be borne.

Later on, almost all the parents told of having thought that they would not continue to participate in the group. The group transference was so intense that even the leader had the feeling of not being able to bear the situation and to fear that the container might be shattered – leading him, too, to feel that the experience might soon be interrupted.

The group containment continued, however, and at the end of the first meeting, we witnessed a change in the group's state of mind and the beginning of contact among the participants, with exchanges of practical information and telephone numbers in the event of a need for instructions or advice about nutritional or therapeutic strategies.

Soon, in the following sessions, the impact of the onset of diabetes on the life of the couple and on the child's education began to be discussed. Also spoken of was the parents' risk of being hyperprotective of their children, almost as though they were taking their places in the administration of therapy and limiting the children's opportunities to get themselves out of the difficulties of everyday life on their own, ignoring their need for autonomy. Together the parents discussed their reactions to the children's initial requests to spend a few days away from home, sharing their perplexities about these requests to be alone while studying or on vacation over the summer. In fact, it has been pointed out how much the presence of a chronic illness and the necessity for treatment can influence the achievement of adolescent autonomy (Seiffge-Krenke 1997).

In the group, the parents took responsibility for their difficulty in accepting that their children were detaching from them and in an indirect way for accepting that they were becoming responsible for their own therapy. Recognizing how important that was, though difficult, helped them not to fear emotional separation from their children, facilitating their autonomy. A measure of the work that the parents had accomplished was the fact that many children, during the following summer, spent time away from home; all of them managed well, and in the course of those experiences there was no hypoglycaemia nor any hyperglycaemic episodes.

This early trial opened the way to other, similar ones that were directed at children and adolescents with various medical conditions other than diabetes – severe obesity, phenylketonuria, rare diseases, or functional somatic disturbances. The accumulated experiences, shared in supervisory groups, allowed the shaping of a culture of group activities that were applied in different ways according to need. When our group of colleagues was ready to launch group experiences directed to children and adolescents, these were always supported by a parents' group, which was conducted at a reduced frequency in parallel with their children's experiences. This solution proved to be very versatile and useful, becoming almost the usual way of working in our group.

Groups with Children and Adolescents

The direct experience of group functioning in basic assumptions and in work groups was very useful to us in doing a quick read of the changing situations that evolved in a progressive or a regressive way, following the emotional fluctuations that invariably occurred in the various groups we conducted. The experience we undertook pushed us to venture into areas that were always new, such as that which will be described in what follows: a group of preadolescents who had been hospitalized for various kinds of somatic expressions that were assumed to have an emotional origin (see the chapter on functional somatic disturbances).

This group would meet weekly for a period of 1 hour, 45 minutes, while once every 3 weeks, the parents, at the same time, would meet with a colleague. In a room that lent itself to this usage, there were several chairs, a box of toys, writing materials, and an individual folder with paper and pastels – basic materials for each child. At the first meeting, the number of children present was only three, which in a short time became a core of six, who adapted over time to the arrival of new participants.

The leader introduced himself and talked about the timing and frequency of the meetings, reminding the participants of the reasons why they were there and that these related to the problems that had brought them to the hospital. He then outlined the main rules, which consisted of the fact that they could talk about anything, but they were not allowed to hurt themselves physically or to put themselves into a situation of real danger. Then he moved on to the introductions by the participants.

"I am Filippo. I had a heart problem, and I came to the hospital since the doctors didn't understand anything. I went back there and began talking with a psychologist, and now I am here."

"I am Gabriele. My parents separated, and now I am here."

"I am Armando. I went to the hospital because I have a headache."

After a period of silence, they asked what was inside the folders and began to use them. Filippo took his; Gabriele gave one to Armando and then took his own. They opened them and one boy sat at a big table, another stretched out on a rug, and the third sat nearby at a little table, turning his back to the other two. Then they began to draw. Gabriele finished first and began to explore the contents of his folder. Armando closed his folder in an orderly way, and Filippo continued to draw. After they had all been silent for a while, the leader asked if they wanted to tell about what they had drawn. Gabriele said he had drawn the sky with two bolts of lightning and some confetti. Armando had drawn three creatures, three "humanoids": incarnations of "faith," "ignorance," and "intelligence."

Filippo had written, "Go to school," because he didn't like going to school. Gabriele said that he didn't like it either because it was boring. Armando was indifferent about it; he had to go to school and so he went, though he didn't like physical education class. The latter statement struck Filippo, because for him that was the only fun class.

Their attention then turned to the box of toys, and they asked if they could play with its contents. Filippo said they might play "bang jumping" (bungee jumping), a game in which a person hurled himself into space, and at the end, before touching the ground, there was an elastic band that would stop him from falling.

The leader brought to their attention that perhaps beginning something such as what we were doing was a little like throwing oneself into a void, and maybe they were asking if there was an elastic band that could prevent them from hurting themselves.

Filippo said that school was like this: "You go in and you go to the back, then when the bell rings you're saved." Armando confirmed what Filippo said; at school you got tired, but he decided to get others to do the talking, those who were older. For him, the difference from elementary school was that recess was shorter, and you couldn't go into the other classrooms.

After talking about school, they asked what their parents were doing; at that moment, they were meeting with another doctor. After saying that they thought they met more often, the boys began to talk about the relationship that each had with his parents. Filippo recounted that they sometimes discussed unimportant things, such as what to eat, but the day afterward everything got changed around. Armando said that he, too, experienced things getting broken; to give an example, he wrote on a piece of paper, "Mom, I love you" and then tore it up.

Gabriele, in the meantime, timidly took a rubber ball from the basket of toys, tied a piece of string to it, and began to throw it and then retrieve it. This seemed to be a kind of "spool game," similar to the game that Freud (1920) – having seen his grandson throw a spool tied to a string outside his vision, then beam with joy when he pulled it back – described as an attempt to master the mother's absence.

Filippo, who was watching, said that Gabriele's game was like bang jumping. Armando, almost as though to detach himself from the emotional content of what was happening, said that it seemed to him it was called "bunging jumping." Then he pulled out some "Magic" cards that he had brought with him, looked at them for a while, and put them back in his pocket.

Filippo remembered having played a game of this type at a house in the country. He had piled up some straw and wanted to throw himself onto it from a certain height, but his grandfather stopped him. Then he discovered some elastic bands in the box of toys. He tied them together to form a kind of catapult, a "weapon" to which he added a paper clip and which he directed toward Armando, asking, "Do you have the Magic cards?"

Armando declared that the "weapon" wouldn't work because there were too many elastic bands, but at the same time he moved behind a table to protect himself. Gabriele, too, protected himself by using the cover of the box of toys as a shield, while he tied a ball to a string to throw it here and there – first toward Armando, then between my legs as though to explore that space. Gabriele was satisfied with his way of having tied the string to the ball, even though it didn't hold and the ball frequently came loose. He accepted Armando's advice about how to tie it to the ball in a better way. "He can't tie it because it's too soft; you would have to move the string from one part to the other."

Filippo said that he could have managed it, while he played with other paper clips that he had found to make a kind of necklace that reminded him of a snake. The session ended with various attempts to establish connections and ties, more or less firm ones, between the ball and other objects, using various materials that allowed detachment but always retained control.

It was surprising that in this first session, in contrast to what typically happens with individual sessions, the boys had already managed to speak directly about the wish to weave together relationships and about the fear of losing them – the fear, that is, of losing relationships with meaningful people and the desire to reconstitute them, as happened with the ball tied to a string.

In this first session, they seemed to be already immersed in topics that would be addressed in the three years of the group's duration: detaching from the parents of their childhood, particularly the mother, while at the same time maintaining a connection. All of them seemed to have felt at ease in the group, whose state of mind – an assumed basic dependence – Armando had represented by drawing the character of "faith." Even though he didn't seem to really trust it, he had brought into play the function of thinking. He expressed a fear of contact in the drawing with the unformed knot of what could represent deep anxieties. The characters of "intelligence" and "ignorance" completed the picture, leaving the understanding of their meaning to the group at a later time.

The boys seemed to have given themselves a great deal to do to establish connections, immediately announcing that the problem was that of "throwing (or hurling) one's self." From the beginning, they asked the question of how they could be connected to each other and how to keep hold of the mother's breast at the same time – at bottom having the impression of not being able to succeed.

Puncturing the ball, something that in effect they didn't do, could have represented the wish to "enter aggressively inside the mother," piercing an outer covering to enter into contact with the internal. Hurling things with a catapult could express throwing their own states of mind out into the group in a nonverbal way, through action, reaching the others directly with their own emotions, waiting to find a vocabulary to be able to express them in words.

Very rich material developed with the arrival of new participants, deepening the complexity of emotions, the ambivalence of the participants' feelings, and the need to maintain a connection even under the pressure of aggressive impulses and particular trigger points. The various basic assumptions, the struggles, and the pairings alternated with each other, reappearing with a continuity that permitted getting to know them and leading the group more frequently into the modality of a work group. In this group, too, at a certain point the anxieties were turned outward: elastic bands, strings, and paper clips were used to protect the therapy room from potential invaders. Over time those objects left space available for fantasies, dreams, and thoughts.

The group agreed to live something that they hadn't been able to experience: entering into contact with their own feelings. Especially because it is not easy for preadolescents to express in words what they feel, the group represented a significant learning experience for them – a place in which they could learn to express themselves and perhaps think something that earlier had not reached that form of expression.

In addition, the function of the therapist in the group was not aseptic; transferential and countertransferential elements were sometimes particularly intense. Adequately managed, these elements represented an aid to the understanding of the group's emotional life. The therapist, participating in the group's states of mind, had also experienced emotions that they had allowed him to access and that in that moment the participants were feeling.

Moments of transformation and of completed passages followed. A unique moment was a session in which it was necessary to communicate to the others that a parent of one of the participants had been lost. The long silence, the compassion, the setting aside of conflicts and friction in order to express to the bereaved person the other participants' nearness in experiencing this grief together – all these contributed to a reliving of the large and small developmental episodes of grief that had marked their lives. Beyond the actual circumstances, there is always a moment in the life of the group in which anxieties linked to death leap out. In effect, as soon as a group comes into being, it experiences a fear of dying and other anxious emotions that are generally set aside but that re-emerge in the course of group meetings, until the point that their working through is possible.

The parents' group, too, became a transformative container that witnessed important changes and gradual awareness. They, too, could confront the various family core problems, and they learned to talk about their feelings. This allowed them to reduce the "burdening" of their children, to notice the difficulties that the children had to cope with and, when possible, to identify them within the relationship with themselves – not only as an expression of aggression toward them but also as an inevitable journey – in order to gain distance from the people to whom the children had been most tightly connected, their parents. Almost all the parents recognized having been deeply changed in the course of the experience and having succeeded in seeing in their children things that had earlier escaped them.

The Last Meeting

At the last meeting of a group that had lasted three years, which occurred at around the time of the Christmas holiday, four boys participated who – in contrast to the others – had not concluded the experience by the time summer vacation began. One of these boys brought in a letter of greeting.

All agreed that they felt better and no longer had the problems that led them to the hospital. Alessandra, however, asked herself whether the positive results would be long-term. In her words:

> Now I'm well, my leg doesn't hurt any more, and I'm even rather happy to be completing this experience. But I ask myself what might happen in the future if bad things come back and the group is no longer here?

It's surprising to think how well this girl succeeded in appropriately expressing her contradictory feelings surrounding the conclusion of the experience that had accompanied her over the course of the prior three years. She expressed pleasure at no longer having a fixed commitment that in some way limited her activities during the week, while at the same time, she was aware of uneasiness at starting to miss a relationship with the group that had gone on over time and had given her security. Having acquired these skills, it is probable that, if problems did eventually come up again, it would be possible for Alessandra to mentally cope without the necessity of using her body to express her distress.

"It doesn't come back to me," Carla stated, explaining that "I'm doing well with my friends in high school; they don't make fun of me, and I no longer get headaches." And Andrea added, "My cough hasn't recurred either. I have fun in the group, whereas before I thought I was antisocial."

At that point, the leader said something about the fact that now they were more capable of talking about their feelings and sharing them – something that had helped them cope with *thinking things*, which earlier managed to express itself only through the body.

Looking for something in her purse, Alessandra found a ten-cent coin and started to make it rotate on a vertical axis. Using her fingers, she pressed it into line with the rotational force and observed the duration of movement along the vertical axis, before the gravitational force dropped it to a horizontal position. From this a game was created that, with the addition of two more coins, involved first Carla and then Alessandra. They threw the coins simultaneously to see who could make the movement last for the longest time. It was a joyful game that both of them set about trying to win but with the evident pleasure of being together and sharing this activity. To identify the owner of the coin that sustained movement for the longest time, they wrote the initials of their names on each one and asked each other if they could take them home; after a while, when interest in the game had faded, each retained her own coin.

I doubt that those youngsters knew anything about the etymological origin of the symbol, but I think that they had an experience of a torn ticket or pass that, when united to its complementary part, expressed a meaning that went beyond factual reality. With that game, they had in some way answered the question with which Alessandra had begun the session; the symptoms expressed in the body's concrete, presymbolic language had over time been enriched by an emotional significance that now allowed the attribution to them of a meaning and a communicative modality. The fact of taking home the coin used in the girls' game was not connected to its value of ten cents, but it signified taking home the ability to assign mental value to what had been expressed somatically – in other words, attributing a symbolic value to something that previously hadn't had one.

Almost to confirm how true that was, someone suggested playing the game of "hangman," an old game that at one time children played with paper and pencil but for which these youngsters used an application on their cell phones. In this game, one tries to guess a word by identifying each of the letters that comprise it, with a limited number of attempts, because every mistake made contributes to progress in constructing the figure of a man on a gallows, which when completed means the defeat of whoever hasn't guessed the word.

They had selected a difficult variation of the game: these were phrases suggested electronically, with some internal empty letters. Everyone actively participated in trying to win the game according to strategies that were thought up and shared in the group; the power of thinking helped them overcome many subsequent trials. A couple of times, the group finished "hangman" with the victim hanged, but overall, they shared the satisfaction of having coped with difficult situations and of having done well enough in pulling themselves up by finding the missing words.

Finding the missing words meant giving mental expression to what didn't have it earlier, and it required the involvement of the body, which they had brought to the hospital; through transformative work carried out in the group, they managed to no longer be in a position of need.

Experiences like the ones described convinced us more and more that group psychotherapy is a very versatile tool in health institutions, and we agreed that it must occupy an important place among the therapeutic options offered by health services.

Notes

1   Type I insulin-dependent diabetes is a chronic illness that suddenly manifests during the course of childhood, adolescence, or adulthood. For reasons that are still not understood, the immune system attacks the pancreatic cells that produce insulin, the enzyme that allows sugar in the blood to be transformed into the energy necessary for the body's activities. If the condition isn't treated with adequate medication therapy, a high level of sugar in the blood is produced (hyperglycemia), and the increased

concentration of sugars can over time create problems in peripheral microcirculation, especially in the kidneys, eyes, and feet. Insulin not provided by the organism itself must then be provided externally, in the right quantity, in three or four injections a day, together with accompanying glycemic checks. Also required are the right diet and appropriate physical activity, because if the amount of insulin injected is more than what is necessary, a low level of blood sugar (hypoglycemia) results in a lack of energy for the vital functions, which can lead to a coma; while if it is less than the correct dose, a condition of hyperglycemia is created that over time can lead to well-known complications. In diabetes, the danger of dying and the anxieties linked to it is ubiquitous, and one can eventually die if the prescribed treatment isn't followed, though a sudden coma can also occur due to excessive adjustments.

2   Measurement of glycemic hemoglobin is a laboratory test that tracks the progress of the glycemic level in the blood during the prior three months.

References

Bion, W. R. (1961). Experiences in groups. In *Experiences in Groups and Other Papers*. London: Routledge, 1991.

Cramer, B., Feihl, F. & Palacio Espasa, F. (1979). La diabète juvénile maladie difficile a vivre et a penser. *Psychiatrie de l'enfant*, 22:5.

D'Alberton, F., Nardi, L. & Zucchini, S. (2012). The onset of a chronic disease as a traumatic psychic experience: A psychodynamic survey on Type I diabetes in young patients. *Psychoanal. Psychother.*, 26:294–307.

Fonagy, P. & Moran, G. S. (1993). A psychoanalytical approach to the treatment of brittle diabetes in children and adolescents. In *Psychological Treatment in Disease and Illness*, ed. M. Hodes & S. Moorey. London: Gaskell Press, pp. 166–192.

——— (1994). Psychoanalytic formulation and treatment: Chronic metabolic disturbance in insulin-dependent diabetes mellitus. In *The Imaginative Body*, ed. A. Erskine & D. Judd. London: Whurr Publishing, pp. 60–86.

Freud, S. (1920). Beyond the pleasure principle. *S. E.*, 18.

Seiffge-Krenke, I. (1997). One body for two: The problem of boundaries between chronically ill adolescents and their mothers. *Psychoanal. Study Child*, 52:340–355.

Chapter 12

Anxiety Management Groups for Staff Members

Another contribution that psychoanalysis can bring to the culture and clinical practice of a health institution is its attention to the emotional life of unified work groups, through tools that allow the sharing and working through of the emotional vicissitudes of professionals who work within them.

In our practice, beyond the group interventions devoted to patients and the parents of hospitalized children, described in the preceding chapter, groups dedicated to hospital staff have demonstrated a particular impact when they have successfully connected to the resonances that professional life brings up in the subjectivity of health care workers.

We often have occasion to observe that in health care organizations, traditional training processes are aimed mainly at the acquisition of specific techniques and methods, the definition of protocols, and organizational modalities. An equal amount of attention is not devoted to the emotional aspects of professional life, in terms of productivity and the quality of the relationship with patients. Actually, making room for psychological factors connected to the practice of health care is an important factor in improving clinical practice and in countering the burnout phenomenon, a condition characterized by emotional exhaustion, a sense of frustration, apathy, and depersonalization, which afflicts more health care workers than one might think.

Petrella (2009), speaking from a psychiatric perspective, which can be applied to any other specialized forum, maintains that:

An important tool championed by psychoanalysts-psychiatrists who work in institutions is the discussion of clinical cases in groups composed of various professional sectors that are employed in the therapeutic setting. I think this should be considered the principal way to allow untrained persons as well, through a personal analysis, to gain a view of the clinical case that includes the patient's unconscious fantasies and those of the caregivers. The psychoanalytically oriented discussion group is an irreplaceable tool in institutional work.

DOI: 10.4324/9781003252238-13

Over the course of my professional life working in public entities, I have been involved in numerous phases of health politics; I have seen the rise and fall of ideologies, theories, and cultural tendencies. For example, from a period in which a culture supportive of labour led to calling the hospital an "establishment," there was a shift to a culture that aspired to run the hospital according to the rationale of a firm, and in fact, hospitals are now called "firms."

These differing eras of health culture are united by the attempt to manage changes in various structural set-ups through organizational operations that, even if they significantly change those set-ups, remain culturally ineffective, to the point that the underlying attributes of every organizational reality seem to drag on with their own particular characteristics through a progression of generations of clinicians, apparently without interruption.

In fact, processes of organizational restructuring that I have witnessed or participated in – though at times impacting the directions taken, the number of professionals, and organizational connections – have managed only to scratch the surface of practices within those structures that unfolded and continue to unfold according to codes that could be predicted by modalities in effect that have solidified over time.

One of the traits of a complex organization that immediately leaps out to the non-casual observer is that the various functional realities of which it is composed, even within common interventional protocols, have ways of functioning that are totally specific, as well as operative codes that are reconstructed according to the implicit culture to which they necessarily refer.

Menzies Lyth (1960) – in addition to having helped us understand, in preceding chapters, that professional motivation depends in large measure on the events of the internal world and on the necessity of coming to terms with vicissitudes of the development of individual workers – told us that culture, the structure and way of functioning of work groups, are for the most part determined by the needs of the members to find a psychological balance. In her words:

> The need of the members of the organization to utilize it to counteract anxiety leads to the development of defence mechanisms structured socially that appear as elements of the structure, culture, and ways of functioning of the organization. A social system of defence is developed over time through collusive interactions and agreements, often unconscious ones, among the organization's members regarding the form it will take. The socially structured defence mechanism then tends to become an aspect of external reality with which the institution's old members and its new ones must come to terms.
>
> [Menzies Lyth 1960, p. 443]

In her research on the nursing service in a general hospital, Menzies Lyth identified a series of defence mechanisms at work in health organizations (see the chapter on the basic therapeutic factor).

It is probable that these are manifestations that are in part inevitable in carrying out a very complex job, but if one adds in the frequent manifestation of distance, tiredness, and psychological and physical illness on the part of the staff in a given department, we can imagine that we are confronting something that arises specifically in that situation, one that has to do with the emotional encounter with patients, with the resonance it finds within the individual, and with the functioning of the group to which the individuals belong.

Standards of behaviour originating in the group culture of every effective organization are printed in huge invisible characters at the entrance to each department and are immediately legible to whoever comes into contact with them. Adaptation to implicit rules and to the mechanisms of protection from the anxiety of a functioning reality is required in order to be able to feel that one is fully part of the group; non-adaptation, in fact, sets in motion an imperceptible, gradual slide in marginality or in psychic and somatic suffering.

If the professional task appears to be stamped with a clear rationale, the individual choices that structure it are connected to underlying motivations to which professional choices, often unconsciously, constitute a response, and the acquisition of mature professional competence depends on the result and on "the elaboration of existing connections between personal identity and professional identity" (Senise 1988, p. 218).

It is not always easy or even possible to take meaningful steps toward an awareness that involves a difficult reckoning with childish, immature, sick aspects that we notice inside ourselves. Our professional choices, too, may have originated from attempts to come to terms with the deprived or sick child that we feel we were, the carriers of irreparable deficits that we have registered inside ourselves, or to accomplish a new and different relationship with parents capable of the care and closeness that we would have wanted to have.

If an individual cannot admit to himself the presence of desires that for him are not permissible, those connected to love, aggression, ambition, the need to be recognized and reflected back, he will seek among those in his surroundings someone with particular characteristics, someone well suited to the embodiment of these undesirable aspects. In a work setting, too, apparently conflictual yet stable relationships come into being in this way, because despite apparent incompatibility, they have underlying, hidden identifications through which the subject can be in contact with – and at the same time maintain distance from – his loving desires, his aggression, and his need of narcissistic confirmation through other people who live these parts of himself, expressing them in his place.

That can take shape through a psychic defence mechanism made up of a mixture of concepts of identification and projection that Anna Freud (1936) described in her essay "A Form of Altruism" and that closely relates to "the system of collusion and negation" described by Menzies Lyth (1960). In a psychoanalytic sense, identification consists substantially of a psychological process of rendering a part of the self similar to an admired or hated object, and projection consists of placing into the object feelings, aspects, or parts of the self that a person doesn't recognize or rejects in himself.

Anna Freud noted that some patients, in facing instinctive desires that are unacceptable according to their moral rules, project them onto persons in their environment with whom they actualize an unconscious identification. Through this shift, it becomes permissible for patients to busy themselves with the accomplishment of their desires. This happened to the young governess who, unable to recognize her childhood desire to own beautiful clothes, to marry and have babies, busied herself with the activities of her sisters and their friends.

Although surpassing everyone else in cleverness and receiving accolades and admiration, she developed an extremely modest personality, ready to be content and to demand little of life, except to interest herself with great passion in the romantic escapades of friends and relatives or to dedicate herself with self-denial to the accomplishment of very ambitious projects of the persons who lived near her.

> Instead of utilizing her energy for personal aims, she put herself entirely at the disposition of others, emotionally participating in their experiences. She lived the lives of others and not her own. Her superego, which condemned a particular instinctual impulse when it related to her own ego, was surprisingly tolerant of it in other people.
>
> [Freud 1936, p. 137]

Professional choices related to the treatment of others – this is true of the doctor in a more covert way, while it is more evident with the psychologist – can allow us to bypass recognition of problematic aspects of ourselves and can lead us to take care of parts of ourselves through taking care of others.

The process of personal and professional maturation means that this inevitable initial motivation gives way to more intimate contact with the self and that more primitive identifications and projections give way to more developed defensive, structuring formations; in this way, professional maturation comes to be part of the general process of transformation and growth that unfolds over the course of one's entire life.

We have seen in the preceding chapter that Bion (1961) identified in his basic assumptions the modalities of implicit functioning in which a group is mapped out in the various moments of its life: *fight/flight, pairing,* and *working group.* Although it might seem barely credible, in general, only a small part of the activity of groups operating in various hospital structures progresses to the level of a working group, while the majority of working life is fixed at more primitive emotional levels.

Group Interventions and the Management of Anxiety

As described in the previous chapter, the idea of launching group meetings took shape slowly but progressively, little by little, as we were confronted in hospital practice with the difficulties of working in an environment in which the primary objective was to cure physical illness, and only with great difficulty were connections with concomitant emotional problems recognized, both in patients and in the staff.

The hospital's working model seems to be based on that of acute illness and emergency: that is, a person is in good health and suddenly an external factor, an illness, threatens his healthy state, and he turns to the hospital to provide a restoration of his well-being so that he can be returned home.

This is a basic model in real situations that are urgent and acute in which a skilful and timely intervention permits the resolution of a critical situation. But perhaps one could say that the linear model – crisis, opportune diagnosis, problem-solving action, overcoming of the crisis – is not applicable to other situations, perhaps the majority, in hospital practice.

If we aim to accomplish at least in part a safeguarding of health according to the criteria established by WHO, which defines health as "a state of complete physical, mental, and social well-being, and not the simple absence of a state of illness," the delivery of care, in the hospital as well, must aspire to more complex models. It would be a bit as though, if I draw on rescue procedures as an analogy, the capacity to mobilize lifeboats and evacuation systems were to become a prioritized aspect to which the culture of navigation would be adapted.

In reality, in chronic disturbances, in pathologies of an aetiology not entirely known and that manifest only gradually, the navigation – taking a journey together with the patient to the point of arriving at a secure port – makes up the greatest part of everyday practice, which naturally assumes that, in the case of necessity, the skill and speed would be available to carry out all the emergency measures.

I think that one could say, even at the risk of running up against a degree of oversensitivity, that often in the hospital culture the capacity for thinking, at least for a shared thought that can maintain contact with emotions, does not reach the level of importance that it deserves. And here I am not talking about rational thought or about the extent of scientific investigation that in these settings often reaches the level of excellence; rather, I speak of a thought that can come into contact with what happens inside us and in the relationship with others.

Many somatic pathologies are caused by or coexist with a difficulty in giving expression to what moves along the deepest levels of emotional life, often constricted to a silence without means of expression. Reopening a level of trust and contact with one's own mind means opening new communicative flows that promote more developed states of well-being and at times render the experience of illness no longer necessary.

To give an example, many training initiatives are implemented to make specialized technical abilities – made necessary by new technologies – more accessible to the staff, but if these are not inserted into a context that takes account of a way of applying them to patients, the result is scarcely applied. Indeed, at times, an extreme technique is based on the necessity to cut off all contact with emotions.

Actually, it has been noticed that when meetings with the staff took place, each time that a process of communication was successfully activated and the sharing of emotional contents occurred, very meaningful experiences of change emerged in the way that individuals came closer to their work and in their relationships with patients and colleagues. Group meetings with the staff created the possibility of undergoing and sharing an experience with colleagues such that, even though they might come from different viewpoints, once they had shared similar conditions, they were mutually recognized as attentive interlocutors.

A Concrete Experience

The material that follows derives from a series of meetings of a group formed from the personnel of two staff cohorts of doctors and nurses who, following a merger and reorganization, were unified into a single operational unit (Perini 2006).

From a technical, administrative point of view, the unification of the departments and staff seemed to be effective; in contrast, putting together a single operational group composed of professionals who had matured in different cultures appeared to me to be a very difficult task. It involved raising for discussion the methods that each group had unconsciously constructed to protect themselves from anxiety and according to which each person had, again unconsciously, put together his professional identity. This meant confronting anxieties connected to the loss of a sense of belonging, to a sense of extraneousness, to a fear of indifferentiation (Bleger 1992).[1]

I therefore proposed to the new director that we set up groups with voluntary participation that would meet every three weeks. The group session would begin with the presentation of clinical material by the participants and would allow ample time for discussion – a re-enactment of Balint's groups (Balint 1957; Balint and Balint 1961), adapting them to the demands of the hospital.[2]

Defined by a specific place and time and being directed toward both the internal and the external are features that guarantee the opportunity for group thinking in sharing, metabolizing, and transforming the feelings linked to daily practice and quantities of unworked-through anxiety. These were anxieties that, if lacking access to a symbolic working-through activity and if not integrated into the individual and group psychic apparatus (Kaës 1999), continued to pervade the individual, the group, and the institution as "residuals" (Roussillon 1988), capable of initiating various forms of suffering.

Forbidden elements of methods for protection against anxiety that each structure placed as the cornerstone of its activity infiltrated, like waste materials, the crevices of the institutional structure (Roussillon 1988) – often enclosing themselves there, as though in crypts – and their expressions frequently led to individual unease. In fact, institutions – almost by definition hostile to the establishment of connections perceived as threatening – are rarely able to take care of these aspects or even simply to tolerate within them the presence of individuals who are in contact with their emotions. As a matter of course, the working through of these primitive emotions, confined to the personal dimension, happens in an informal way in "interstitial practice" – that is, in places at the border between the time and space of the working activity (see the chapter on the basic therapeutic factor).

Our attempt, made through a formal group, aimed to create a place where some of those emotions and deep sensorialities could be brought to signification and language – via a process that, in Corrao's (1998) terminology mentioned in the preceding chapter, has been described as a *gamma function*, that is, through the use of what Neri (2001) defines as "the capacity of group thinking to 'metabolize' sensorial elements, tensions, and fragments of emotion that are present in the field."

So this is how a project related to beginning the work groups got underway, groups that pertained to the management of anxiety and emotional dynamics in relationships with patients (and their families) and with co-workers (doctors and nurses). The project was based on the hypothesis that contact with acute pathologies in children exposes health care workers to considerable levels of anxiety and, if these anxieties are not contained or held in check, they tend to bring about the mobilization of defensive manoeuvres in the staff, which has a notable impact in the relationship with our little patients, their families, our colleagues, and with other professionals who collaborate in the treatment process. It was affirmed that these mechanisms of protection against anxiety influenced the work organization as well and that they could lead to non-collaborative attitudes, emotional detachment, adoption of working styles that did not encourage collaboration, and the devaluation of the contribution that each worker could bring to life on the hospital ward.

The initiation of discussion groups that aimed at a global approach to the ill person and at improving the participants' capacity to "know how to listen" to patients and colleagues, involving the whole of the staff in an effective togetherness, tended to promote the creation of a shared working culture and to contribute to the improvement of an emotional climate that supported the recognition of the individual contribution to the work at hand within a shared project.

In the first of a series of meetings that involved all levels of the workers in a particular department, a nurse talked about the situation of a child who in that moment was greatly preoccupying the staff.

> The child, a "preemie" of less than a year, had been hospitalized for resurgent respiratory problems only two weeks after his return home following a period of six months in intensive neonatal therapy. He had some hypothermia, but his symptoms were not as worrisome as the fact that his mother alternated between moments when she seemed close to him and moments in which she distanced herself, almost hiding, and was subject to crying spells.
>
> That night the child was connected to a series of devices that monitored his condition and that often, in merely reacting to his movements, sent alarm

signals without there being an actual dangerous situation. Every alarm caused agitation in both the child and the mother, such that they could not sleep.

The nurses, after having been called by them several times, judged that the child's condition made it possible for him to be detached from the technological equipment, after which the child, entrusted to the mother, calmed down, and both of them could rest.

This episode lends itself to describing the full trajectory of oscillation between the persecutory and depressive anxieties of catastrophic disintegration that circulated in the group. They stemmed in part from the child's condition – since he was in a state of precarious health along the border between life and non-life – and in part from deathly fantasies about the group's functioning. This was a group with viable parameters that loosened at certain moments but that the participants felt as an alive thing, a baby-group struggling to live within the structure, trying to see if "throwing away the equipment" could help protect the baby against the monster of a very persecutory institution.

Group life is closely connected to the experience of death. As soon as a group is born, it is pervaded by death fantasies; from the moment in which it is born, it is exposed to the fear of having to die or of being born prematurely. These fantasies periodically emerge in every group, when the violence of feelings that have been kept split apart interrupts the group's mental space and the group becomes able to recognize and host them. Just as every birth involves pain, so does the birth of a group space that can host thinking. Whether our group might be a living bud or a gem that had already faded was an experiment. At the beginning of each new meeting, it happened that there was a sense of almost incredulous marvel at the fact that the group continued to live – just as each time, at the end, there was surprise at the richness of contributions and the rhythm with which integrating movements were seen to occur (Carbone 2005).

At a certain point, while there was containment of anxieties in the group, the experiences of individual participants were integrated and began to form a shared narrative plot; an intense turbulence appeared on the horizon. Waves of persecutory anxiety resurged without resolution with the intervention of another participant who asked the meaning of what was going on, beginning from the moment that working conditions and relationships within the department were such that the members were not even permitted to know each other. Great personal suffering was borne within the group, suffering that derived from the person's not feeling recognized in his work or at a professional or personal level. He complained about the anonymity of the structure, and in the moment in which he was allowed to express this, he did so in a way that the others registered as an attack. The emotional dimension was overheated, and external factors were called into the field – the organization of the staff, the politics of the administration. The group was divided into favourable and contrary elements.

The fragile vessel of group thinking appeared to be hindered by vertexes of turbulence; the risk of psychomotor disorganization (Kreisler 1981), which could lead a baby-group to death, not sufficiently contained – avoided when the nurses renounced the reassuring protection of technology and entrusted the child to the warm containment of his mother – again arose in the group, which like a little baby found itself exposed to alternating experiences of mortal disintegration and containing integration.

The fact that the group had permitted there to be a very deep decontamination that helped transform feelings of impotence and death into shared memories and solid connections was also illustrated by what emerged in another meeting:

> The previous day, a nurse had greeted the parents of a small child who was unwell and, upon encountering them outside the hospital a little before the group began, asked how the child was doing, to which the reply was that the child had died. The group shared the nurse's emotions and asked whether one could ever get used to the deaths of children, a rare enough event on that ward. The child had been ill for some time and there wasn't much hope, but no one thought she would pass away so suddenly. On the one hand, there was the fact of not having expected it, and on the other, the fact that the death of a child is something to which one cannot become accustomed. Someone said that there are children to whom we become more affectionate, and their deaths cause us more pain.
>
> Someone asked whether it was right, from a professional point of view, to visit the mortuary when a patient dies.
>
> Our culture has found ways to share the pain of loss of persons whom we hold dear. Over time, the trajectory of grief allows the connection with the person to weaken, and we are free to dedicate ourselves to new relationships.[3]
>
> Visiting the mortuary pertains to the sharing of pain.
>
> Someone said that often we try to convince ourselves that we will do better if we avoid contact with situations that we find too intense, but on the contrary, reality tells us that if we can manage to keep in contact with pain and loss, we can share them, all in all finding some meaning in what we do. Many experiences of the participants revealed that, even in situations of children who were lost, the contact with parents was maintained, and the latter had in turn demonstrated affection and recognition toward those who had shared those terrible moments with them.
>
> The group allowed the participants to talk together for the first time about the deaths of little ones that over the years had peppered life on the hospital ward. "Bodies in the closets," for whom the mourning process – which everyone had kept inside without being able to share – thus found a way to be addressed. One participant said, "I'm struck by the intensity of feelings that have emerged in a situation in which, typically, I would tend to slam the door at my back."
>
> There had been an opportunity to talk about anger over the way in which the deaths of some children was experienced and about the tenderness that surrounded those of others. It wasn't true that one suffered more from the loss

of children toward whom one felt more affectionate. The deaths of X and Y, two children who had passed away in recent years, were compared. While X did well during the period preceding death – and this had been a source of comfort and consolation for the parents and the staff, who had a chance to tell him goodbye and to attend the funeral – Y never stopped suffering, and according to some, he had not been helped to suffer less; he had no possibility of experiencing "a good death."

Reliving these events of mourning had reminded the participants of deaths in their own personal stories as well, had put them into a state of emotionally revisiting such events, and in the group there was a continuing discussion about good deaths and bad deaths. The good deaths were those in which the connections were not truncated and it had been possible to complete the work of mourning. Mechanisms of identification had allowed aspects and characteristics of those who had gone to find a place inside their loved ones. In regard to one of these children, one person said, "I remember him with tenderness. At times I still see his mother and we greet each other with affection."

The bad deaths were those in which persecutory monsters came to pull the cover of guilt over whomever was left behind, when the pain and anxiety had ruptured connections with the child, and when there was a feeling of not having done everything possible to help him exit in a serene way or when it hadn't been possible to say goodbye.

An emotional rendering, equally rich, was presented at a subsequent meeting, when a nursing supervisor related an episode that had happened the previous day.

A little girl arrived at the emergency room in critical condition. For various reasons, not one of the many medical advisors who were called would admit her into their better-equipped wards; they came, gave their advice, shared the situation, but as soon as it was concluded that they couldn't admit her, they disappeared.

Continuing her account, the nursing supervisor spoke of a dream that she had had the previous night.

The Dream

She was in the hospital, in a long corridor, probably of a geriatric/rehabilitation ward, when an elderly man fell out of a wheelchair. She approached him to help him get up but couldn't manage because the patient seemed too heavy for her. Her colleagues nearby did not appear inclined to help her; indeed, they maintained that it was her duty to lift him since she was the nursing supervisor; she replied that she wasn't the nursing supervisor of that department and so it wasn't her task.

Then she added that along the corridor (which she emphasized was quite long), there were 27 rooms stretching from the most distant one, which was a paediatric room, to a geriatric one (where she was at that moment) – that is, all the way from new-born babies to the terminally ill. In her associations, she said that she had had the feeling of having to occupy all the phases of life, and to feel on her shoulders "the weight of [all the patients'] life and death."

This woman, because of her character traits, had assumed at this moment in the life of the group the role of "dream bearer":

> These dreamers become dream-bearers due to the effect of the internal neces-
> sity of establishing, by means of the dream, a psychic space that is larger than
> their own and whose limits are extended to those of an other, of more than
> one other, and to a whole group.
>
> [Kaës 2007, p. 168]

The dreamer had dreamed the difficult task of passing from the old modalities of treating patients to the newer and more cumbersome modalities, which she felt the weight of carrying forward.

The beginning of life and its end seem inclined to extremes of a spatial dimension that, in this case, allowed the expression of a contrasting flow of emotions that this woman had felt the previous day in relation to the struggle of a baby, born not long before, to continue to live. They also described the feeling of impotence and the need for support that she had experienced through the dream, which she brought to the group – or rather that perhaps the group had asked her to express.

The Non-dream

Almost to confirm this intuition, another colleague who was interviewed afterward said that she, too, had dreamed the previous night, and even though she said she didn't remember what the dream was about, she reported having had agitated sleep.

The Non-sleep

In the subsequent meeting, another group member related that usually, when unpleasant things or things that worried him happened in the hospital, for him to go to bed at night was almost a protection. He tended to go to sleep immediately, as though he wanted to postpone his troubles until the next day. This time, however, he told of having had disturbed sleep after some difficulty in going to sleep.

In this intense exchange at the beginning of the meeting, the emotions experienced during the previous day and relived in the *hic et nunc* of the group dimension seemed to have reached a possibility of being recognized and shared in a modality of narrative, participatory expression. Each in his own way, all the participants took home something of what had happened in the hospital, particularly the anxiety tied to the feeling of having been left alone to have to care for a small child in serious condition. That was mixed with a worry about taking care of a group that lived and proceeded with difficulty within the institution and of a leader who would have preferred to be more directly involved in the activity.

Different degrees of figurability – of the possibility, that is, of transforming feelings and primitive emotions into mental representations that were potentially shareable – had served as a vehicle toward signification through the representation of the shared dream, the repressed dream, and the disturbed sleep. We learned and shared over the course of the group's experience the experiential truth of the function described by Bion (see the chapter on therapeutic factors). We talked about children and we talked about the content of the anxieties that circulated in the group. The concept of containment and restitution of what was anxiety-provoking seen with a new-born is important not only for mothers but also for persons who work in a health care system or other social setting and who have to deal with other people who are suffering.

More often than one might imagine, anxiety and the worries of patients reverberate in the mind and body of those who take care of them. The identification of tools for them to be adequately worked through is necessary so that the vital capacity of continuing to dream will not be compromised, during sleep or during waking hours, in our personal life and in our professional activities.

Participation in group activities was not unanimous. Not all those who began attending meetings continued to come to them. Perhaps an experience so loosely connected to hierarchical logic and reasoning exposed them to too many anxieties of disorientation or depersonalization. A consistent and stable core was formed that made up the framework of the experience, and the work of the group, like a pebble of meaning thrown into a sea of non-thinking, was transformed into waves of resonance and empathic sharing that could reach even very distant institutional and interstitial places.

Notes

1   For the loss of elements of a combined sociability – that is, of those elements of indifferentiation present at any level of personal and group development that are unconsciously deposited into the group.
2   These groups, called "Balint" for the name of the analyst who theorized them, are composed of about ten participants who meet weekly on a regular schedule to discuss clinical situations brought in by the participants in turn. The meetings focus on the way in which the clinician experiences the relationship with the patient and are held in an atmosphere of examination in which value judgments and criticisms are reduced to a minimum, in such a way as to broaden the experience and the possibility of understanding patients' problems.
3   In this regard, see Neri (2002) on the sharing of pain.

References

Balint, M. (1957). *The Doctor, the Patient, and His Illness*. London: Churchill Livingstone, 2000.
Balint, M. & Balint, E. (1961). *Psychotherapeutic Techniques in Medicine*. London: Routledge, 2001.

Bion, W. R. (1961). Experiences in groups. In *Experiences in Groups and Other Papers*. London: Routledge, 1991.

Bleger, J. (1992). *Symbiosis and Ambiguity: A Psychoanalytic Study*. London/New York: Routledge, 2012.

Carbone, P. (2005). *Adolescenze, percorsi di psicologia clinica [Adolescence: Journeys in Clinical Psychology]*. Roma: Magi.

Corrao, F. (1998). *Orme. Contributi alla psicoanalisi di gruppo [Footsteps: Contributions to Group Psychoanalysis]*. Milano: Raffaello Cortina.

Freud, A. (1936). *The Ego and the Mechanisms of Defence*. Abingdon, UK: Routledge, 2018.

Kaës, R. (1999). *Le teorie psicoanalitiche di gruppo*, trans. A. Verdolin. Roma: Borla, 2006.

———. (2007). *Linking, Alliances, and Shared Space: Groups and the Psychoanalyst*, trans. A. Weller. London/New York: Routledge, 2018.

Kreisler, L. (1981). *Clinica psicosomatica del bambino [Clinical Psychosomatics in Childhood]*. Milano: Raffaello Cortina, 1986.

Menzies Lyth, I. (1960). A case-study in the functioning of social systems as a defence against anxiety. *Hum. Relat.*, 13(2):95–121.

Neri, C. (2001). *Gruppo [Group]*. Roma: Borla.

———. (2002). La condivisione del dolore [Sharing pain]. *Quaderni di Psicoterapia Infantile*, 44:8.

Perini, M. (2006). *L'Organizzazione nascosta. Dinamiche inconsce e zone d'ombra nelle moderne organizzazioni [Hidden Organization: Unconscious Dynamics and Shadow Zones in Modern Organizations]*. Milano: FrancoAngeli, 2015.

Petrella, F. (2009). Psicoanalisi e psicoterapia in psichiatria: storia e prospettive di un rapporto difficile [Psychoanalysis and psychotherapy in psychiatry: History and prospects of a difficult relationship]. Paper presented at Bologna Psychoanalytic Center, March 28.

Roussillon, R. (1988). Spazi e pratiche istituzionali. Il ripostiglio e l'interstizio [Institutional spaces and practices: The storeroom and the small space]. In *L'istituzione e le istituzioni [The Institution and the Institutions]*, ed. J. Bleger, E. Enriquez, R. Kaës, F. Fornari, P. Faustier, R. Roussillon & J. P. Vidal. Roma: Borla, 1991.

Senise, T. (1988). Elaborazione delle motivazioni profonde e consapevolezza delle possibili inferenze di esse e della "weltanschauung" nella relazione come requisiti indispensabili nella relazione terapeutica [Elaboration of deep motivations and awareness of their possible inferences and of "weltanschauung" in the relationship as indispensable requisites in the therapeutic relationship]. In *Il Lavoro clinico con gli adolescenti: atti del congresso [Clinical Work with Adolescents: Actions at the Congress]*. Paper presented at the University of Padua, Department of Pediatrics, November 24–26.

Chapter 13

Group Sessions with Volunteers

On Books and Reading in the Hospital

At times a contribution to our understanding of the emotional dynamics underlying our own activities is required of voluntary service organizations as well, in particular those that play a direct role with hospitalized patients – in this case, hospitalized children and their parents. Organizational frameworks, shaped according to the rules of civil code and inscribed in registers established by laws governing voluntary service, operate in quite a varied way within hospital settings, often bringing invaluable contributions via their activities or in promotional work, sensitization, support, or the collection of funds. Often they are organizations of hospital patrons, family members, or sympathizers who recognize themselves in the statutory goals of promoting and teaching the rights of the persons whom they represent.

Among the contributing organizations that operate within the hospital is *Bibli-os'*, an association that promotes the diffusion of books and reading on the wards, in the same vein as similar experiments found in other national and foreign clinical settings. Since its inception, Bibli-os' has been devoted to the value of experiences that are already present and the relationship with other similar realities; it was born and launched within the hospital setting. In the words of its founder, Ilaria Gandolfi, Bibli-os'

> intends to support young inpatients and their families through reading, thereby creating a space of mental and actual escape at the same time, as only a book knows how to do, thanks to its little papery windows into fantasied worlds. It is the desire to alleviate the suffering and loneliness of those who live out a hospital experience that has inspired us to develop Bibli-os', a library service available to all patients and their family members.
>
> [www.Biblios.it 2017]

Of fundamental value in their initiatives, the organization places profound faith in books and in their worthiness in transmitting messages of love and life and in children and their strength to overcome difficulties. To that is added the hope that a good public hospital might gradually become less detached from the emotional or cultural reality of arranging a journey to treat the disease, which might also be a journey of the individual's growth and well-being.

DOI: 10.4324/9781003252238-14

In recent years, the Bibli-os' organization has succeeded in accomplishing most of its objectives, lending or reading books to children and parents in hospital wards, as part of an intervention coordinated with health care workers in the various settings in which it operates. Its extremely valuable presence is by now part of daily life in some departments, with a level of activity that can't be ignored – that is, they have reached the point of lending 18,000 volumes to hospital wards over 7 years.

Bibli-os', by its own definition, wanted to move about "on tiptoes" without interfering with medical or nursing interventions or with the role of parents. It wishes to offer children and their parents relational moments connected to books and reading, utilizing parts of the day in which charitable activities are not taking place. The activities of Bibli-os' have included both lending books and making available reading experiences with trained volunteers.

Reading, writing, and enjoyment of all the other modalities of artistic creativity are among the tools that humanity, since its inception, has devised to preserve experiences – finding meaning in them and providing security when facing the external world, the internal world, and their indomitable instinctual forces. Just how much reading can lend itself to alleviating suffering and emotional pain was brought home to me by Enrico, a nine-year-old boy. For a long time, his internal world had been pervaded by intolerable sensations connected to the experience of loss of affective relationships with his love objects – loss that could be imagined as having constituted an originary trauma. Over time, he had managed to work through those sensations and to find the words with which to define the state of mind that he described as falling into something anxiety-provoking that he wasn't familiar with. However, this had cost him a great deal in terms of development, because in trying to master those anxious emotional states through repetitive actions, it became difficult for him to feel as though he were like his companions or to feel interested in many of the activities of children his age.

Enrico imagined that relationships were not secure and that to establish ties with someone almost inevitably gave rise to a "story," and so he would call up a fantasy that led him to think that, in the end, he would inevitably fall into a canyon of loneliness and sadness. Over time, the story took a less tragic course, and at times he could imagine that a calmer future awaited him.

In one session, he told me that:

> There's a book that I like a lot because it talks about what my life is like, because you know that I fight all the time with my dad – that my dad says I'm crazy because I have fits, I'm possessed and it isn't possible to be possessed by fits forever. This book talks about things like what happens between me and my dad. The boy in this book is real, and some authors have told his story, and he doesn't know why he became famous. You'd like to buy it too, right? My mom read the first few pages to me, then I read it because I understood it was the right book for me. The boy used his imagination, and I too imagine

ideal places – all of them beautiful, like I want them to be, as I would want them to be.

When I told Enrico that it seemed marvellous to me that something that had happened in his life was similar to something that had happened to others as well, he answered: "You're right – I found them in the book. I like it because it's as though I. . . . Anyway, it tells something about me. But there are only a few kids like me, special kids."

Thus, a book allowed Enrico to identify with a boy who became a special man and didn't feel that he was merely "crazy, awkward, possessed, different." I then became curious about the book and bought a copy. It was *The Dreamer*, by Pam Muñoz Ryan and Peter Sís, and it told of the life of Neftalì Reyes, a "strange" boy who as an adult became the Chilean poet Pablo Neruda, winner of the Nobel Prize for Literature. To my young patient, the book was useful; even if it were useful only for him, it would have been worthwhile for the book to be written. The intense anxiety that Enrico expressed in his behaviours, as happens to many other children, gave rise to states of mind that were pervaded by intense and painful feelings, almost unimaginable by an external observer.

A written text, stories, fables, are gifts of love. Authors, who are particularly gifted people who can dwell in emotions and intense states of their own unconscious experiences, manage to give them a shape that offers readers the possibility of refinding themselves in it and utilizing it to give words to events in their own internal worlds, in turn. Often this has a reparative function (Segal 1952), reconstructing the relationship with one's own primary love objects that, for one reason or another, might have been deficient and about which regret ends up interwoven into the fabric of the artist's existence.

This function is fulfilled by fairy tales, for example, as Bettelheim (1975) tells us. In every phase of life, children deal with fears, fantasies, and wishes found in the fairy tales that interest them. The stories with happy endings aren't very interesting; it's those in which threatening situations appear, cruelty, dangers, that hold greater interest for children. They don't introduce new elements, though they provide the opportunity to represent emotions that are already there in the child. The story of Little Red Riding Hood, for example, through the character of the wolf, allows expression of fantasied themes tied to the oral phase in which the child relates to the environment through the mouth by licking, biting – and experiencing, beyond the effects of his love, those of his own aggression as well. This is something that can scare him: the possible disappearance or destruction of caregiving figures, invested by him with the intensity of his ambivalent impulses. In fairy tales, through projective mechanisms, displacement, and transformation of active into passive, his own aggression gets diverted toward something external – for example, the wolf – and getting away from it is enough for him to feel secure, liberating the relationship with the parents from all its disturbing affects.

In this way, fairy tales and stories permit those who read them to recognize instances of overcoming difficult situations and conflicts of existence that all of us inevitably face – often beginning with the early phases of life, when the nodal points of sensorial experiences occur at a presymbolic level, before or beyond the capacity of thinking with which to represent them in images.

Early on, Freud (1908) emphasized the connection between the experience of childhood play and artistic creativity, maintaining that every child, when playing, can be considered a poet, from the moment that he constructs a new world based on the demands of his internal world and in a real temporal dimension:

> Mental work is linked to some current impression, some provoking occasion in the present which has been able to arouse one of the subject's major wishes. From there it harks back to a memory of an earlier experience (usually an infantile one) in which this wish was fulfilled; and it now creates a situation relating to the future which represents a fulfilment of the wish. What it thus creates is a day-dream or phantasy, which carries about it traces of its origin from the occasion which provoked it and from the memory. Thus past, present and future are strung together, as it were, on the thread of the wish that runs through them.
>
> [pp. 147–148]

This text conveys the thinking of early Freudian theorizations, when the psychic apparatus was imagined as divided into "psychic provinces" of the conscious, preconscious, and unconscious, with strictly monitored borders in the form of censures that we can imagine as frontier guards, armed with the defensive mechanism of repression that can allow – or not – the drive contents to take root in consciousness. Through a transformative activity, then, narrative or artistic creation allows the content of an instinctual wish to reach consciousness in changed forms, thus escaping censorship and repression.

In the subsequent development of psychoanalytic thinking, traumatic elements were seen to date back to fault lines in an early relationship that compromised the basis of the sense of self. In a dimension located at the dawn of psychic experience – where, often in sensorial form, the possibility of "thinking thoughts," of symbolizing, or of achieving representative mental activity had been placed at risk – creative activity, as occurs in dreaming, came to be considered a way of transforming those emotions into narration capable of expressing the rupture of the relationship with the object and the attempt to recover it.

In more serious cases, just as in the life of any ordinary person, the written word and the word that is read represent powerful tools with which to express chaotic emotions, charged with attraction and longing, which once transformed into shareable artistic forms can permit their users to be in contact with those sensations and to share those experiences in an attenuated way.

The hospital is frequently occupied by children who experience events that undermine the sense of continuity of their own existence – children who are lost in a forest of therapeutic procedures that are often painful and incomprehensible to them, who encounter monsters and powerful enemies against whom they don't know how to defend themselves, and who at night, helpless, can be attacked by a threatening presence, and they fear being run over by emotions too strong to manage or even to express in words.

Hospitalized children can be greatly helped by learning from books that, before them, someone else has overcome these obstacles and by knowing that the possibility exists of escape from the forest and of finding the way home, which in the end is made possible by perseverance, diligence, and shrewdness, all brought to bear in order to find unexpected solutions with which to face the dangers and the monsters – even if this is only a way to accompany them on their journeys and to make them feel that they are not alone when reality seems to preclude a happy ending. Perhaps the first request that children and their parents make to those who care for them on an emotional level is to be helped to understand and share the intensity of emotions that they are dealing with at this moment in life.

We have seen in the chapter on communication of diagnoses that an awareness of this has led health care workers to modify their way of communicating diagnoses over the years and to attune medical and psychological attitudes to the necessity of fostering maximal comprehension by children and their families. Beyond what professionals can do, artistic expressions, literature, and poetry offer tools with which to give words and images to the emotions that human beings experience when negotiating life passages and while undergoing the various phases of growth or of interruption of disease, pain, or grief.

An American researcher, James Pennebaker (1997), demonstrated that written elaboration of one's own emotions and one's own thoughts, in some situations, can be an effective health-promoting tool. Applying his writing technique to healthy people resulted in fewer medical visits. In health situations having a medium level of seriousness, various research results have shown improvement in respiratory parameters in asthmatic patients, a diminution of symptoms reported by subjects with rheumatoid arthritis, and better post-operative courses in various surgical pathologies. Research by colleagues at the University of Rome, "La Sapienza," found a considerable improvement in the metabolic equilibrium in patients with untreated diabetes in comparison to control cases (Pastena et al. 2007).

Meetings with the Group of Volunteers

Aware of the fact that emotional factors could influence their way of working and their relationships with children and parents, as the activities progressed little by little and new queries were put forward, the group of volunteers gradually noticed the need to initiate meetings in which it would be possible "to face up to each other about the experience on the ward." On a voluntary basis, the Bibli-os' group participated in these meetings, as did nursing and medical personnel who included the head nurse, the director of the unit, and psychological consultants.

In an endeavour that lasted some years, the themes discussed were multitudinous. There was a steady, gradual increase in the group's awareness of the influence of emotional factors seen in individual volunteers and in the group as a whole. With a frequency at first monthly and later bimonthly, on the day and at the time agreed upon, the group came together without a precise agenda for the day. Each participant could suggest a topic for discussion – an episode from his work that was close to his heart and that he wanted to call to the attention of others. The only rule to be followed was that, in each meeting, someone took on the task of writing up a verbal synthesis of the themes that had emerged, which would be read at the next meeting, and over the course of the group's progression this led to a thick file of documentation.

The written record often presented an occasion on which to marvel at the quantity and depth of the themes discussed, which – although organized into the tracking of activities that involved both individuals and the group – almost disappeared from the conscious memory of the participants. "But did we really say these things?" was a question that frequently came up when reading the report of the prior discussion reopened memories that had apparently been forgotten but that were firmly anchored in the deepest area of functioning.

In the course of the meetings, we often saw an oscillation between dedicated attention to administrative aspects of the organization and the relationship between volunteers, the administration, and other corporate structures and the creation of conditions such that there could be an emergence of emotional aspects connected to the relationship with young patients, their parents, and the various pathologies that characterized them. One began to realize that, in the group as well, wanting to stay in contact with topics that had involved the people in the group on an emotional level coexisted with a need for some distance.

Personal Motivations and the Activities of Volunteer Organizations

Volunteer organizations constitute an irreplaceable resource within health care institutions. Their work varies from promotion and from socialization of individuals about the health and social conditions of the categories of people whom they represent, to a necessary trove of resonance with their needs for improved services for them, to the collection of economic resources with which to provide endowments and missing equipment or to integrate treatment teams with new professional resources.

In most cases, organizational life allows transformation of pain connected to the presence of pathology into an activity of high social value, which permits doing something to improve the conditions of the people whom the various organizations are concerned with. At times there is an implicit risk that in the organization's activities, shared defence mechanisms will also be activated with respect to the reality of the pathology, based on denial, projection, and an attitude that underlies neediness and dogmatic attitudes that divide administrators, professionals, and entire sectors of social reality into "us good ones" and "the others, the bad ones" – that is, those who don't understand the sacrosanct rights of the persons whom the organization helps. An example of that is the observation that only in some especially virtuous settings do the various organizations pool their resources in order to contribute together to the realization of more general objectives. It is more common that every organization pursues its own specific objectives for the protection of its members' rights.

For Bibli-os', too, the necessity of reflecting on the motivations of individual volunteers and their organizational activities has been apparent. Monthly groups, beginning with the concrete experience taking place on the ward, has allowed volunteers to be able to talk about their way of experiencing the activity that the organization proposes, of confirming its choices, or, at times, of raising for discussion some of the behavioural modalities.

One of the first and most important topics put forward was that of the volunteers' emotional involvement in the lives of persons whom they encountered in their activities. This was especially the case when they ended up establishing particularly intense and/or problematic relationships due to the child's or young adolescent's need to involve volunteers in their affective problems. A recurring question pertained to how to behave with that particular little boy or that particular little girl who seemed able to access a delicate area in a volunteer's sensitivity. In other words, how to find an appropriate dimension between maintaining detachment, on the one hand and accepting involvement without it becoming excessive, on the other?

One volunteer, for example, related that her motivation to participate in the reading initiative had been her love for children, but from the time of her initial involvement, she had noticed that she was overidentifying and "taking home" all the problems of the children whom she met on the ward. Considerable time was needed in order for her to realize how much this made her suffer, and it was only having been able to share her difficulties with the group that had allowed her to reflect on her motivations and behaviours, eventually leading her to find a more balanced way of relating that permitted her to make more realistic interventions, ones that were more helpful to the persons whom she encountered. At other times, the subject of discussion pertained to the irritation that became apparent for some of the parents who did not allow a relationship with their children or who did not seem able to see how much the child enjoyed sharing a moment of meeting.

As we have seen in the preceding chapters about professional choices, deciding to participate in a volunteer organization's activities can also involve an implicit need, such that, beyond providing help to persons who turn to them for aid, there is a hidden benefit, a form of fulfilling a personal need. It is as though, through deep identification with the recipients of one's own activity, one can listen to and be in contact with personal aspects that are difficult to recognize in one's self and of which we may not be aware.

On the other hand, reading itself represents a specific experience in which written words by someone who has observed the necessity of giving a form to personal contents are employed to encourage an emotional experience in someone else, in a chain that unites the reader with the writer. If the idea of writing is born of a need for "eternity" – i.e., to fix a moment in the incessant flow of time – this is indistinguishable from the need to relate to others. At bottom, what inspires modern man to create or to enjoy cultural experiences is not so far from what led primitive man to paint on the walls of the caves of Altamira – in some manner "writing" his experiences, thereby preserving them in a way that has challenged time.

Perhaps no writer could write without imagining, more or less knowingly, at least a potential reader, a person who could appreciate his work. The reader in turn renews the connection with the writer who is on the same wavelength with parts of himself that resonate with what he reads. For the reader, too, there is a need to be read by the book, to find a listening for emotions whose writer has allowed them to assume a shape. Writing and reading seem to have an underlying common need to be listened to. If the need to find an interlocutor capable of listening or of giving shape to the formlessness of the events of our internal world is the basis of the communicative act that unfolds between writing and reading, putting oneself forward as an organizer of reading and listening can also imply the wish to be listened to, just as one listens to children to whom one suggests reading.

The extremely valuable activities proposed on wards where there are children with various illnesses and parents in difficult situations presuppose that an overly intense identification with children who need to be heard will be avoided. That is, there will be an avoidance of the risk of excessive emotional involvements in situations that lead to confronting existentially difficult scenarios. To have been able to speak of these things in the group, sharing similar experiences, was felt by the participants to be of extremely valuable assistance to them as they continued to generously provide their services, without being overly drawn into problems that went beyond the help that could be given in such situations.

Reading to Infants

Another important topic that was discussed was the possibility of opportunities to suggest reading experiences to babies, even those under a year of age. These activities are promoted by some organizations – with the support of ministerial boards as well – such as "Born to Read" (www.natiperleggere.it), with the aim of promoting reading in early infancy, which is very ingrained among doctors in key roles and in hospital settings.

Often, in the face of rejecting attitudes or incomprehension regarding their suggestions – on the part of parents who maintained that the baby was too little – the volunteers asked themselves what might be the sense in suggesting such a reading experience. In reality, these proposals were not aimed at transmitting specific narrative contents as much as they were suggestions for brief moments of relationship for the baby, during an empty period of his day, thereby involving him in a multisensorial and preverbal modality in which sound, gestures, words, and narrative structures provided the picture of a safe environment. This modality of approaching a baby sometimes involved the family, too, in an activity that could benefit the relationship.

This is not a therapy or an "educational" intervention as much as it is a pro-posed "tiptoe-ing," according to the spirit of Bibli-os', toward participation in an interaction in which emotional contents, through various sensorial and percep-tive channels, formed a "protonarrative envelope" (Stern 1995). This "envelope" introduced meaningful experiences through a narration endowed with coherence and capable of utilizing diverse modalities. Everyone will have seen a book for babies who don't talk yet, constructed of material that facilitates experiences in which touch, vision, smell, movement – all unified into the voice of the person reading – offer the baby experiences of sensorial integration. In its preverbal aspects, in fact, the voice precedes contents and thoughts, and – through percep-tual outlines (visual images), conceptual ones (symbols and words), and sensori-motor ones – comes to constitute ways of representing the experience of "being with another."

One thinks that children are able to perceive with every sensorial modality the qualities of expressive human behaviour, of representing them abstractly and transferring them into other modalities. Stern's (1995) hypothesis is that, at a preverbal and presymbolic level – and thus beyond all awareness – the connection between different perceptual modalities may produce a sensation of familiarity and a sense of continuity of experience, where what happens in a given moment and what has already been experienced are located in relation to each other. This permits the child to construct an integrated experience of self and others, starting from the first weeks of life. The same process of integrating perceptions con-tributes to the formation of the "sense of self," with the impetus of "affective attunement," a fundamental experience whose presence or absence determines the quality of childhood relationships.

Golse (Golse and Roussillon 2010) speaks of three levels of preverbal narrative: *sensorial narrativity*, which is expressed in the register "of being"; *behavioral narrativity*, which plays out especially at the dyadic level, in primitive connec-tions between mother and baby; and *verbal narrativity*, which precedes the advent of narrativity of the word in its strict sense.

Roussillon (2015) accurately describes the processes of the birth of mental experience, illustrating moments of primary and secondary symbolization (see the chapter on the birth of mental experience). This is the process through which everyone constructs representations of their own experiences in the world, tran-scribing early sensorial, affective, and motoric experiences at different mental levels – experiences that are structured around the parent-child relationship, the fundamental relationship of subjectivity.

Lullabies, books for children – what meaning might they have if not to give shape to children's sensoriality and early anxiety-provoking experiences, within a relationship that gives them a repetition invoking security? To these processes, experiences such as that of Bibli-os' can add small moments that have value in themselves, without the pretext of being problem-solving or exclusive in shar-ing an experience with children and parents that can take on the most varied meanings.

Interculturality

Additionally, entering into a relationship "with what is different," with parents who come from other countries and other cultures, held a noteworthy place in the questions posed by the group. Besides simple misunderstandings due to rudimentary knowledge of the language, there were moments of non-communication and of difficult relationships with persons who came from other cultural and social frameworks, even though in general the experience of meeting proved not to be especially problematic. In some cases, volunteers found themselves facing requests, excessive demands, or even expressions of aggression that created problems for the people who, at that moment, had turned to those persons with respect, tact, and delicacy. Some members of the group had had earlier experiences in the field of immigration, and this helped them understand that apparently demanding and aggressive behaviours can characterize persons who have experienced – or who have subjectively perceived – previous situations of discrimination and reacted to them impulsively. It was noted that when one placed the child and his needs at the centre of the intervention, a way could easily be found to resolve the parents' misunderstandings as well.

The Relationship with Health Care Personnel

In some cases, group meetings allowed health care personnel to share some of the emotional problems pertaining to the relationship with seriously ill children – for example, in cases in which critical-care situations absorbed the workers' thoughts. A specific case was evident when the personnel was emotionally involved in a death that had happened a few days earlier. An especially silent attitude on the part of some of the nurses was read as an indication of something that didn't go well in what the volunteers were doing. However, those and other situations in which a change of attitude on the nurses' or doctors' part due to a functional overload that poured down on them at times, making them less available, were also sometimes interpreted for what they were. Opening channels of communication and sharing states of mind led to overcoming unrealistic attributions of intentionality; these could be seen from an alternative perspective once fantasies and projections were exchanged – promoting, in contrast, greater comprehension and greater closeness.

The work of health care personnel and of volunteers was also united by reflections on attitudes of increased neediness on the part of the parents, who asked health care institutions to fulfil educational roles that, at some junctures, the family seemed to have renounced. More and more often, one could observe the influence on the ward's functioning of an emotional climate that became more and more typical of our times – in which it seemed that one could not impose rules on children – and that the family's educational function had been delegated to other entities, to the school or the health care institution. The group's reflections allowed them to take into consideration how moments of difficulty, such as those connected to a hospital stay, can accentuate these problems. At times when it was necessary to establish rules, it was useful to be able to propose them in a calm way, remembering that a rule always has two sides – as happens in the moral of a fairy tale, when it is said that "you can't do this," followed by the message that "if you do that, you'll avoid getting into trouble."

In conclusion, an important function of regular group meetings was that of offering a "trove of resonance" for feelings and states of mind that are born of the encounter between the volunteer's motivation for an intervention and the concrete reality that clinical practice puts forward.

References

Bettelheim, B. (1975). *The Uses of Enchantment: The Meaning and Importance of Fairy Tales*. New York: Vintage Books, 2010.

Bibli-os' (2017). Riunioni mensili Bibli-os' e personale sanitario [Monthly meetings and health care personnel]. U. Pediatra d'urgenza e pronto soccorso pediatrico. November 2014 – March 2017. (Publication for internal use.)

Freud, S. (1908). Creative writers and day-dreaming. *S. E.*, 9.

Golse, B. & Roussillon, R. (2010). *La naissance de l'objet*. Paris: Presses Universitaires de France.

Pastena, R., Tabasso, C., Pepe, L. Maida, P. & Solano, L. (2007). Effetti della tecnica della scrittura sul benessere e il controllo glicemico in soggetti diabetici con diversi livelli di alessitimia [The effects of writing technology on well-being and glycemic control in diabetic subjects with various levels of alexithymia]. *Psicologia della Salute*.

Pennebaker, J. W. (1997). Writing about emotional experiences as a therapeutic process. *Psychol. Sci.*, 8:162–166.

Roussillon, R. (2015). An introduction to the work on primary symbolization. *Int. J. Psychoanal.*, 96:583–594.

Stern, D. N. (1995). *The Motherhood Constellation: A Unified View of Parent-Infant Psychotherapy*. London: Routledge.

Concluding Reflections

A book undergoes a developmental journey that unfolds over time like a living organism. Life experiences impact the author's sensibility, activating creative functions and causing him to conceive a narrative project. A sort of pregnancy follows, with its happy moments and the fears and worries that it can assume in he who writes, as well as painful somatic expressions.

In the end, the book is born; it enters the world and lives its own life, walks on its own legs, beyond the author's intentions.

This book, too, has had a time of conception and a time of writing, lasting eight or nine months.

During that period, many things have happened.

First of all, the initial project included a list of arguments that, once they were developed, proved too extensive to be fully elaborated in a single volume.

From that came the first surprise, regarding the quantity of information and main experiences in relation to what had been imagined, with the consequent necessity to leave for another occasion arguments that it would have been preferable to include in this book.

In an indirect way, the considerable quantity of work that had been advanced was confirmed, often scarcely perceived from the outside, by me and especially by the people who collaborated with me.

Another important moment was the sharing of the contents of various chapters with those directly involved: the persons with whom the experiential journeys and treatments described in these pages were carried out. For ethical reasons, I considered it paramount to ask their authorization for the publication of events that pertained to them, even though I had changed their names, personal characteristics, and profiles in the text.

This phase of the work, which was imposed on me as necessary for reasons of confidentiality, proved to be quite different from an administrative task.

Meeting people – parents and sometimes children who had by now grown up – and allowing them to read the texts that pertained to them proved to be a gratifying and very precious experience both for me and for them, even though at times it renewed contact with a painful past.

DOI: 10.4324/9781003252238-15

I never received a refusal or a critical note – only a request for minor modifications of episodes that had not been correctly represented or the change of a fictitious name to a more preferred one.

It was like again taking up an interrupted discourse and noticing how much those experiences had been important, still present in people's lives and having contributed to giving them a more calm existence. The same thing happened with the organizations whose activities were described; they recognized themselves in what I had written and found that the foundational values of their activities were respected.

For me, too, those meetings were enjoyable and enriching, and they confirmed how much what I had tried to write possessed a validity and a consistency that was maintained over time. A comment expressed by more than one person authorizing publication was that they were glad their experience could be useful to others.

Between the time that this book was first thought about and when it was completed, many things have changed in my professional practice as well; I have concluded my experiences in the hospital and have dedicated myself to private activities.

Aware that more time is needed by health care institutions to consolidate working practices that view body and mind in an integrated perspective and that my colleagues who participated in the experiences described have yet to cope with great difficulties to fill this gap, while simultaneously going forward in their in-depth, patient daily activities, I hope that this book represents a shared memory and a tribute to their work, whose values and contents will endure – as they have endured in the persons who shared these experiences with us – in order to construct a new phase in which the seeds that have been dispersed may bear new fruit.

Index

For Product Safety Concerns and Information please contact our EU
representative GPSR@taylorandfrancis.com
Taylor & Francis Verlag GmbH, Kaufingerstraße 24, 80331 München, Germany

www.ingramcontent.com/pod-product-compliance
Lightning Source LLC
Chambersburg PA
CBHW050644280326
41932CB00015B/2781